JOIN THE MOVEMENT!

JUNK FOOD FIT

Learn about

Weight Loss, Weight Gain,

Meal Prep, Macros,

...and More!

VISIT
JUNKFOODFIT.COM
TODAY

JUNK FOOD FIT

By Professor Cookie

www.JunkFoodFit.com
@JunkFoodFit

blael books
Junk Food Fit
Professor Cookie

Chief Editor: Wesley Nichols
Copy Editor: Lianny Nuñez

The author and management team can be contacted for permission and inquiries through the website www.JunkFoodFit.com

Publisher's note: This publication is intended to provide readers with information only. It is sold with the understanding that the author, publisher, and group holders are not aiming to provide medical, psychological, or any other professional services to readers. If such assistance is required, services from a doctor or other licensed professional should be sought.

Author's note: While this book is based on factual information and is meant to help others deal with weight and food questions, the content must not be taken as finite commandments but more as informative anecdotes. Not all situations can be dealt with in the same manner, and every weight loss journey should be dealt with on a case by case basis, considering all aspects of the entire scenario. Consult with a doctor before starting any new food or exercise regimen.

Disclaimer: Subject matter is simplified for understanding, although still valid and truthful. For more information and detailed explanations, refer to the sources listed in the back of this book.

The institutions of Penn State University, Montclair State University, and Mondelēz International are not affiliated with the production of this published work, and the information and ideals presented in this book may not be reflective of their own.

Published in the United States by blael books.
ISBN #978-0-9897715-4-2
Version 1.1

TABLE OF CONTENTS

Dedication

Dedicated to all of you who wish for a *better you!*
We are all capable of amazing things,
and I hope to provide you with the right tools
to reach your amazing goals.

Author's Note

With so many self-proclaimed nutritionists and dieticians in the world today, you have to be careful who you listen to when it comes to your health and the food you eat. It's even harder to sift through the thousands of fitness trainers all over social media for the one that will work best for you.

You have to remember, one person's body can be completely different from another person's body, so what might work for one particular fit chick or hulk dude might not work for all of their beloved followers, and most importantly for *you*. Try to find an expert: someone who has been working in the field for years and has trained on that particular topic. When it comes to trained experts, they know how to look at a situation, assess all aspects of the situation, and develop a plan of attack based on all pros, cons, and possible variables.

With that, it is also important to note that advice from trained professionals is not always fail-safe. Sometimes it comes down to personal trial and error, taking the information that is provided by the professional and applying it to your personal situation so that it benefits you and potentially *only you*.

As for me, I'm not saying that I am the number one expert in the world on food and fitness, but I can tell you that I graduated at the top of my class with two degrees in Food Science from Penn State University, I work full time at Mondelēz International as a food scientist formulating new cookies for the world to enjoy (you can thank me for Red Velvet Oreos—oh and Cinnamon Bun and S'mores too!), and I also work part time as a professor at Montclair State University in the Nutrition and Food Studies department. I hope that shows to you that I have a little bit more than enough experience to help you navigate your way through the building blocks of food.

In writing this book, I wanted to create a short guide on food to help individuals understand what they are eating. With all the options out on the shelves today, even I find myself having trouble deciding which bread to buy or which can of soup is healthier for me. Not only do you need to know how to navigate the food and ingredients, but you have to navigate certain marketing methods that are used to trick you into thinking one thing is healthier for you than something else. Lastly, I also hope to clear up a few misconceptions about the terms "processed", "natural", and "healthy" foods. In the end, it's not about pointing fingers at certain foods and saying "eat those" "don't eat that", it's about giving you the knowledge to be able to think on your own and to make better decisions.

JUNK FOOD FIT

CHAPTER ONE

Junk Food Fit

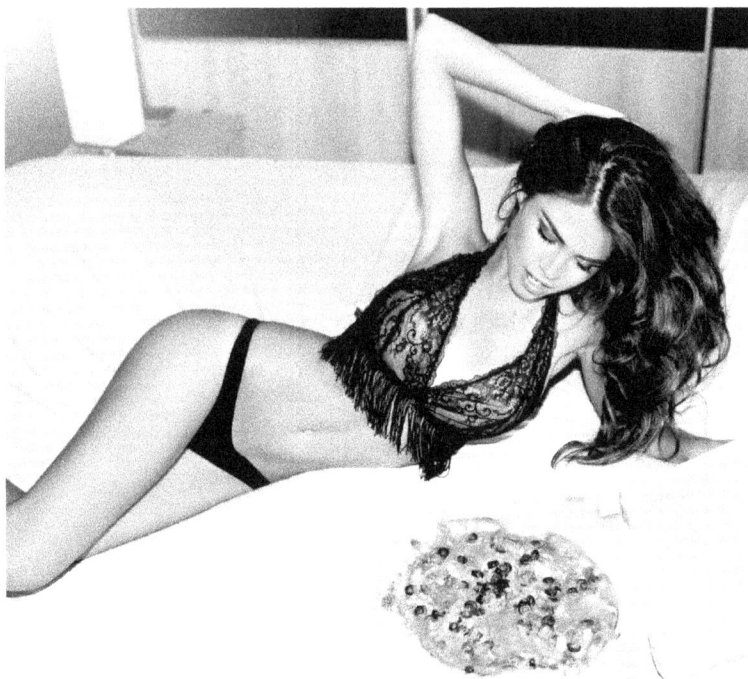

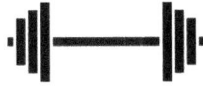

C urrently, I work for a cookie company where I **must** eat five or ten cookies in a day for work purposes sometimes. This is completely separate from the junk food that I may have wanted to eat for dessert or a treat after my workout (mmmm cookies, cakes, donuts, ice cream yum yum).

For me, I **need** to be able to include junk food in my everyday diet, or else I would never accomplish any goals, and eating those five cookies during one 30-minute meeting would have me feeling guilty all day.

By altering my mindset and using the knowledge I have gained over years of schooling and working in the food industry, I have been able to work on myself, my body, my diet, and I have been able to become **Junk Food Fit**.

My lifestyle change to a healthier me was not a "quick fix." The picture on the left was at one of my heaviest periods in my

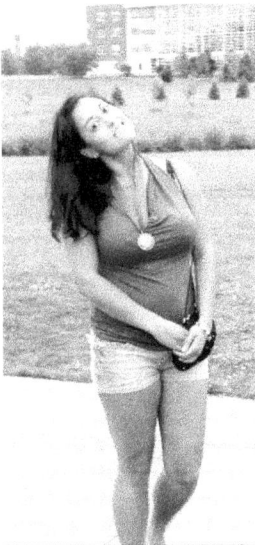

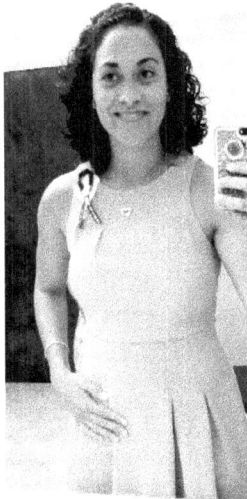

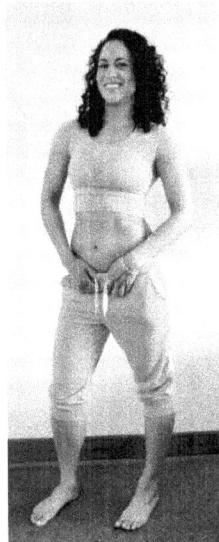

life in 2010, transitioning from college to full-time employment. The middle picture is of me after years of working on my body and adjusting to my busy career life, developing and fine-tuning the Junk Food Fit program based on my own experiences. The last picture is present day—losing the "last 10 pounds" by way of the Junk Food Fit program, counting calories and macros, but enjoying cookies and pizza and burgers on occasion.

Overall, I started at around 175 pounds (although I never used to weigh myself back then), size 13 pants, size large in shirts, and a size 32J bra. Yes, that's right; I said size J. J is a size. Years later, I managed to get down to 137 pounds, size 4 pants, size small in shirts, and a size 30DDD bra.

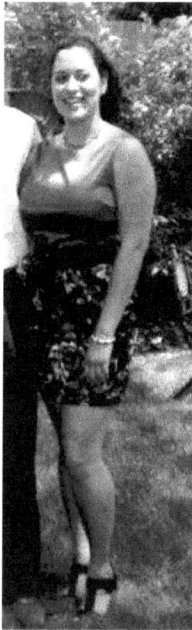

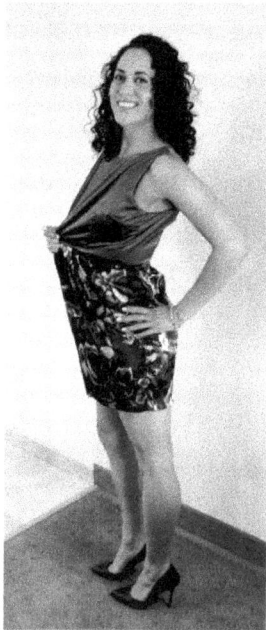

Before
175 lbs
Size 13 pants
Size 32J bra

After
137 lbs
Size 4 pants
Size 30DDD bra

I'm not going to lie and say it was easy—because IT WASN'T! Experimenting with food and fitness on my own and using the concepts behind this very Junk Food Fit program allowed me to completely transform my body. As I learned about my body and about how different foods affect how I feel, I have become that much stronger physically and also mentally.

One thing I need to emphasize is that not only is it necessary to control your diet when trying to lose weight, but also exercise nearly every day is crucial. This book focuses on the food aspect of weight loss and an overall healthy lifestyle, but the best choice you will ever make is to get off the couch and **be active**.

It really doesn't matter what workout plan you follow or which personal trainer you choose. Anything that gets you moving is better than nothing. For me, I love weight lifting—no ladies, lifting heavy weights does not turn you into a man! If anything, lifting weights makes you curvier and definitely more confident—which is the sexiest type of girl you can be!

While "losing the last 10", I kept track of my meals and my workouts. I was in the gym six days per week, weight lifting every day. After the first few weeks, I boosted the program's effectiveness by adding cardio to my routine. My cardio routines varied depending on my mood, but the elliptical was my favorite (burpees my least favorite)—anything to get my heart pumping!

All in all, while the theme of this book is "Junk Food Fit", this doesn't mean you can sit around eating candy bars and playing video games all day. When you get down to the core of your daily routine, Junk Food Fit is a mindset that allows you to **fit** foods that are typically considered **junk** into your meal plan without feeling guilty.

In order to do this, you must be able to **take control**. Pay attention to what and how much you are eating—don't eat mindlessly. To help you with this, I will present you with some food basics so you can begin to understand exactly how certain foods get from farm to table, providing you with essential tools to help you make smarter meal choices.

Throughout this book (and in the courses offered by Junk Food Fit University on our website), you will be presented with simple facts about the food you eat.

As you read, consider the THREE EASY STEPS that the concept of Junk Food Fit revolves around:

STEP 1

Understand - pay attention to what you are eating and what you are putting in your body. Mindful eating is important in both the amount of food you are consuming and also the *types* of foods you are consuming. Be smart and get educated! (Reading this book is a great start!)

STEP 2

Keep track - implement your learnings from Step 1 and track your meals each day. *Use worksheets in back of book*. Whether you are counting calories, macros, or just using a food journal to stay focused, keeping track is the only way you will begin to recognize how much food is too much, not enough, or just right *for you.*

STEP 3

Enjoy - eat all your favorite foods! Just remember that you can't eat them every day, and you can't eat the whole bag of chips—just one serving will do. Let's face it... life's no fun without a little flexibility, so go on and enjoy those treats every now and then!

Another thing to remember when reading this book and while beginning your fitness journey is that no two people are the same. Your journey to Junk Food Fit will be different from your neighbor's which will be different from their best friend's. You will work through those exact THREE STEPS from above, but you may experience them at different rates. Also, you will all encounter the same THREE PHASES throughout your journey:

PHASE 1

Lose weight - in this phase, you need to *keep track* (remember Step 2) of what you are eating. The process will get easier as you go, and you will learn how different foods react with your body, which ones to stay away from, and which ones to eat more of.

PHASE 2

Maintain weight - once you reach your goal weight, Phase 2 is where you begin to eat just enough food to maintain your weight, but not enough to gain any weight back. You will continue to *keep track* of your meals so you can learn how much extra food you can eat now that you are no longer trying to lose weight but aiming to maintain instead.

PHASE 3

Enjoy weight - after Phases 1 and 2, you now have enough knowledge to stop keeping track of every little thing you eat. However, you need to remain conscious of the foods you choose and how much you are eating. Maintain your weight by eating similarly to how you were eating in Phase 2, but you now have the flexibility to live life disconnected from your food journal.

As you live through each of these three Phases, recognize that the journey is a marathon not a sprint. Take as long as you need to fully experience each Phase. Once you reach Phase 3, while you don't need to track everything you eat, you should not use this as an excuse to start overeating and returning to old habits. Yet, we are all human and end up off track sometimes. If this happens, start back at Phase 1 and redo the process. (Sample meals are shown in Chapter 10 and the full Junk Food Fit 12+12 Meal Plans are available through our website for each of the Phases in case you need somewhere to start.)

Using the Junk Food Fit program, I only hope you have the same great results as I did! One last tip though: ***Don't get discouraged!*** There were definitely times when I gave in, binged, and wanted to quit the whole "healthy thing," but then I brushed off, got back on the horse, and kept going! You can do the same... it's definitely worth it! ☺

CHAPTER TWO

Mission: #CookieJar

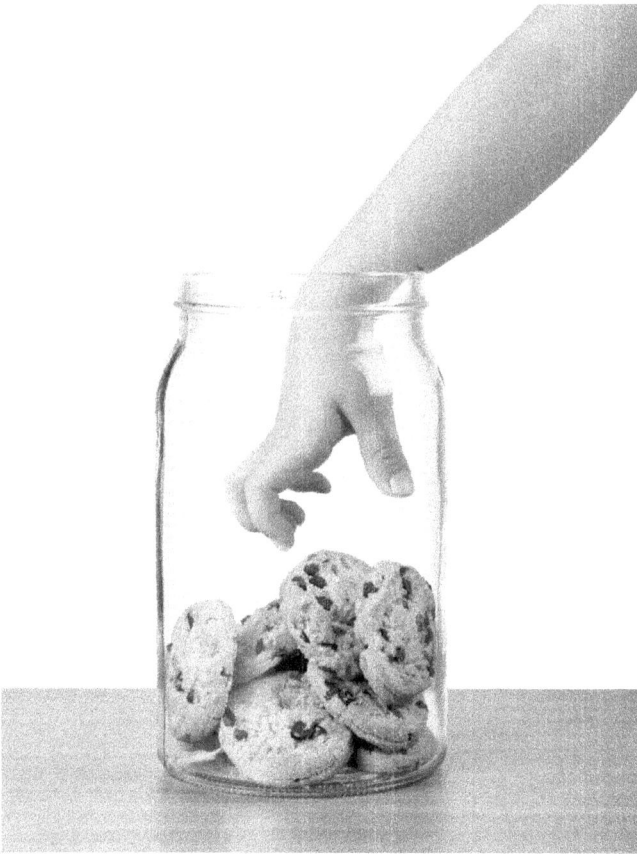

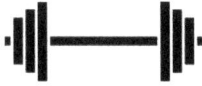

L osing weight is a process. And understanding the food you eat is just one part of the process. When trying to decide between the various apples, juices, steaks, hamburgers, toaster pastries, and popsicles available to you, you should think about the people behind the product and the package (the people involved in making it and packaging it for you), as well as the multiple steps required to take the product from pasture to home. You should take time to understand that milk comes from cows, juice comes from fruits, and flour comes from plants. Understand that the food you eat is part of a larger picture. It is part of a grand industry called the food industry, and the main purpose of that industry is to try its hardest to feed all those who need to be fed.

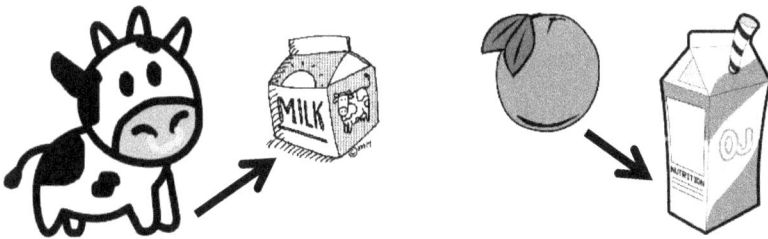

When you think about nutrition, food science, and the food industry as a whole, you must first think about the history of food and how far we have come as a society. Some things that *now* must be learned in a classroom were once commonplace to generations before us. Parents of Baby Boomers come from a time when everyone canned their own peaches, jammed their own grapes, and smoked their own salmon. During the week, they only ate food to survive and to give them enough energy to work; then on the weekends and special occasions, cookies were home-baked and bottled soft drinks were purchased only as a "special treat."

Over the generations, however, the things that were mandatory for a young woman to know before starting a family of her own were no longer handed down to the next generation. Mothers started to work outside of the home, fathers became house husbands, and children spent more time on their Nintendos and computers than in the kitchen or in the garage with their parents.

Lives became more hectic, leading to the concept of fast food and the need to eat on-the-go. Back in the day, consumption of calories was controlled without even trying; nowadays we have the luxury of inexpensive snacks and quick treats, making it so simple to overeat and very difficult to lose weight.

Of course there are some households nowadays that still have retained this knowledge of food. However, just because they know how to can and jam, this doesn't mean that they know the science behind it all. Do they know the pH that is necessary to inhibit bacterial growth? Do they know the names of the bacteria that are typically used in yogurt making? Do they know the reason why grapes break down and form a jelly-like jammy appearance?

While some might know that it's important to keep chocolate at a consistent temperature in order to prevent bloom (the white stuff that appears on your chocolate bar after melting and rehardening), others just throw out the chocolate thinking it's moldy. And more often than not, these same chocolate-trashing people know to place a piece of bread in the cookie jar with baked cookies to keep them from going stale only because "that's what their mommy used to do."

One hundred years ago, my relatives were eating cheese that they made in their own kitchen. Today, I eat cheese that I buy at the grocery store. My relatives used to can and jam fruits to make them last longer than the typical harvest season. Now I can buy fresh fruit in the produce aisle any day of the week all days of the year.

Those hundred years between my great-grandmother and me, that's where the food industry comes in. Over the last century and some, our society has overcome the Dust Bowl, the Great Depression, two World Wars, and many an economic crisis. Along with that, we have greatly increased the efficiency of food-making and created new technologies, advancing our agricultural capabilities in order to supply enough food to feed our nation's ever-growing population.

Looking back, at first the mission was to make sure everyone had enough food to eat. Then the mission became reducing waste byproducts from those agricultural processes, recycling and reusing when possible.

Now the mission, *my mission*, is to Bring Back the Cookie Jar. I want us to go back to a simpler time when mother and daughter cooked dinner for the working fathers and sons. When grandma taught granddaughter how to crack her first egg to make brownies for the grandson's birthday. I want us to go back to a time when mom made her famous chocolate chip cookies and kept them in the cookie jar, stuck a slice of bread in there to keep them soft, and slapped her children's hands every time they grabbed for an afternoon snack (that would surely ruin dinner!). If we go back to a time when sweets and high calorie foods were only consumed on special occasions, not only would our wallets thank us, but our bellies would too.

We need to stop depending on pre-packaged foods and chain restaurants so much, and we need to become self-sufficient in the kitchen. Make your own lasagna, bake your own cookies. That way—*and only that way*—we can control exactly how much sugar goes into the dough and exactly which fresh ingredients we use in the mix.

In reading this book, I hope you learn a little something about food. I want you to be able to take this knowledge and apply to your everyday life; go to the grocery store and understand why one package of bread might be better than another. I want you to gain the courage to step into the kitchen (if you haven't already), and make food for yourself, ultimately changing your lifestyle and potentially losing weight along the way.

Learn about what you eat; don't just taste what you eat. Harness this knowledge, and join the mission. Let's *Bring Back the Cookie Jar* together! #CookieJar

CHAPTER THREE

That's Bad for You!

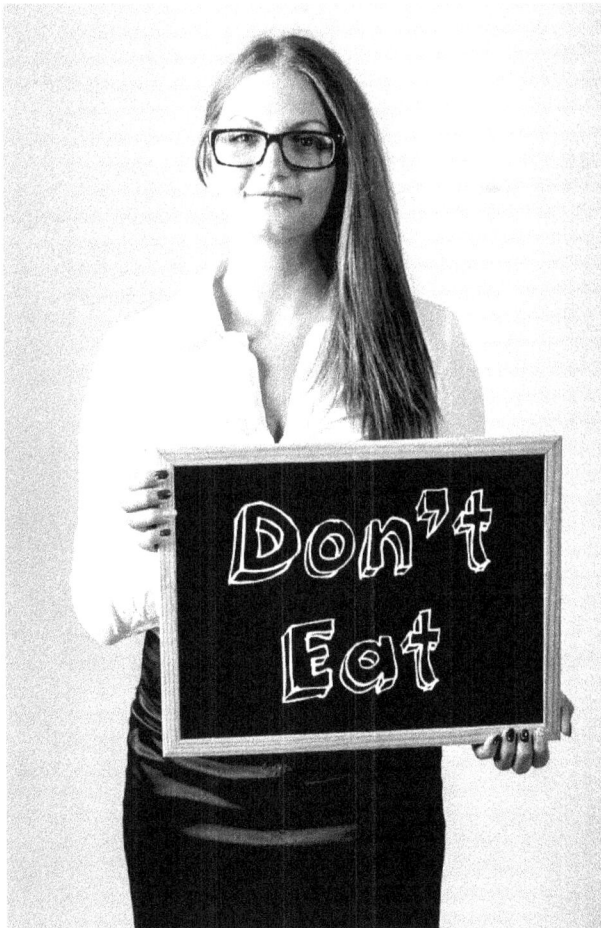

People everywhere have been lectured about which foods to stay away from and certain foods to eat every day in order to "be healthy" (whatever that means). It seems that everyday the advice on the "good" and "bad" status of foods changes. From what you know (and without thinking too hard about it), which is better for you? *Orange juice* or *soda pop*? Now compare the two products using their nutritional facts:

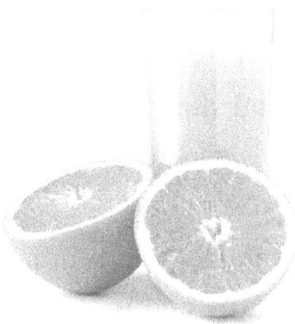

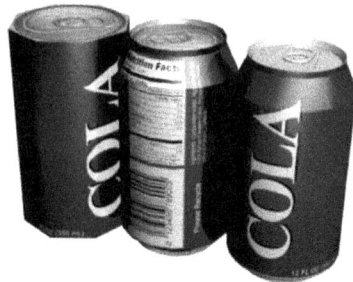

8 oz Orange Juice	8 oz Soda Pop
110 calories	100 calories
27 g Carbs	26 g Carbs
0 g Protein	0 g Protein
0 g Fat	0 g Fat

By solely comparing the calories and carbohydrates, both products are comparable. However, someone might argue that the soda pop is actually better for you because it has fewer calories and carbs. Someone else would argue that the numbers aren't different enough, and that the orange juice is still better for you since it is from a "natural" source and provides you vitamins and minerals. But who is correct?

what does "bad for you" really mean?

Since the dawn of time the phrase "don't eat that it's bad for you" has been synonymous with food products like donuts, candy bars, cupcakes, and fried food (and soda pop). Not until more recently has that phrase been used to refer to foods like white rice, white sugar, and milk. For some fitness enthusiasts and calorie counters, bad foods might even include fruit juice (no matter how fresh) and bread (no matter how whole). For those fitness enthusiasts, eating giant 400-calorie protein bars and piles of peanut butter is a normal day, but an outsider looking in can't comprehend how those same fitness enthusiasts lose weight by eating six meals a day.

To the layperson, it can be confusing and difficult to understand what types of food are healthy and what foods are truly bad for us. One thing you must grasp before anything else is that "bad for you" can mean different things to different people. Also, while one food might be "bad for you" in one aspect, in another light it could be "good for you", all depending on the circumstances.

Take eggs for instance. For the longest time, people have been told that eating egg whites are the way to go and that eating too many whole eggs is bad for you (because the yolk contains too much fat and cholesterol). The understanding was that the fat and cholesterol in the yolk raises blood cholesterol, potentially leading to high cholesterol and heart disease. The problem though, is that by throwing away the yolk—and only eating the white—you are throwing away a ton of good vitamins, minerals, and protein. New studies have shown that eating one yolk a day in conjunction with those egg whites has no effect on blood cholesterol and will ensure you consume those necessary vitamins and minerals like vitamin A and DHA.[1,2]

So in terms of whole eggs being "bad for you", if you look at it one way, you can see that *multiple* egg yolks a day could add too much cholesterol to your diet. Yet looking at it another way, you can see that *one* egg yolk a day could add high quality vitamins, minerals, and macronutrients to your diet.

Aside from the confusion of eggs being good and bad for you at the same time, another example is coconut oil. One of the newest trends in food is using coconut oil for cooking and baking instead of regular vegetable or canola oil. If you look at it one way, coconut oil can be considered "bad for you" since it contains high levels of saturated fats, which increase blood cholesterol levels and could lead to heart disease. Looking at it in another way, however, coconut oil can be considered "good for you" since those saturated fats are *medium* chain fatty acids (instead of *long* chain fatty acids).[3,4]

Studies have shown that the length of the fatty acids have an effect on how the body breaks down and utilizes the fats; the medium chain fatty acids break down faster and have been shown to aid in weight loss, under certain circumstances (this will be explained further in the Fats chapter).[3,4]

Different foods can also be good and bad for you at the same time depending on **who** is eating it and **what** that person's **personal goals** are. For those fitness enthusiasts who lose weight by eating lots of food, they look at food as fuel, and they tend to decide on a food based on the macronutrients that are provided. To them, even though fruit is "good for you" since it provides lots of vitamins and minerals, they might consider it "bad for them" because it contains too many carbohydrates. Likewise, fresh beef steak might be good for *you* since it is a great source of protein, but to *me* I might consider it bad since the fat content is too high.

To answer the first question that was posed: which is better for you, orange juice or soda pop?

The answer is NEITHER.

You can't simply put a label on a food and say, 'This is Good For Every Person Who Walks On the Earth." ***The "goodness" of a food is dependent on the individual***. Genetics, mindset, and personal fitness goals must all be considered when labeling a food "good" or "bad."

While the orange juice is good because the sugars and carbs come straight from the fruit itself, it is bad because all it provides is carbs (no protein or fat). And while the soda pop is high in added sugars (which some people consider bad), it is good to some because it provides energy in the form of caffeine and is in fact fewer calories than the orange juice.

In the end, it all comes down to two concepts: *moderation with consistency* and *discipline with variety*.

Moderation: everything can be eaten; there are no good or bad foods. It's all a matter of the circumstances, time, and place.

Consistency: you should remain consistent with a few aspects of your diet to create a regimen. This includes number of calories, macro goals, and specific meals that stay the same throughout the week. You should plan ahead and prep your meals; DO NOT care about what other people think!

20

Discipline: even if only for a few weeks at first, you really should count calories—not only calories, but macros as well. Counting your intake of proteins, carbohydrates, and fat does take dedication, but the results are worth it. Too much or too little of one macronutrient could throw your diet and weight off-balance.

Variety: let's face it; we all get bored eating the same foods every day. Variety will help you stay focused by adding inconsistency to your consistent meals. Even if it's as simple as switching your snack every day—apple, orange, kiwi, banana, there are so many to choose from—the small bit of variety can make all the difference!

Okay, you caught me! These two concepts overlap a little, leading to just *two* key words that you should always remember: ***variety*** and ***consistency***. Whether you are trying to lose fat, maintain weight, or build muscle, you must remain consistently focused, adding sprinkles of variety not only to your diet but also to your workout routine.

Comparison of Foods (Good vs. Bad)

Some examples of similar foods and how they can be seen as both good and bad

Cow's Milk
Good: Protein, vitamins A&D
Bad: Lactose (if lactose intolerant)

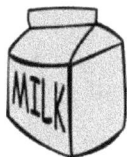

Almond Milk
Good: No lactose, low calorie
Bad: Low protein, few vitamins

Regular Peanut Butter
Good: Good quality fat, high protein
Bad: High fat

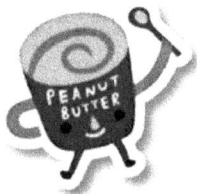

Low Fat Peanut Butter
Good: Good quality fat, high protein
Bad: Higher in carbohydrates (added sugar)

Turkey Burger
Good: High in protein
Bad: Animal product (if vegetarian)

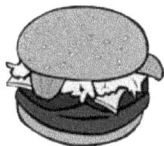

Tofu Burger
Good: High in protein
Bad: Soy product (controversially linked to cancer)

Coffee
Good: Caffeine for energy, considered "natural"
Bad: Digestive irritant

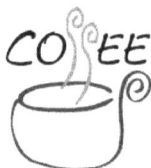

Zero Calorie Energy Drink
Good: Caffeine for energy, contains B vitamins
Bad: Artificial sweeteners

Hummus
Good: Good combo of macros
Bad: May be higher in fat

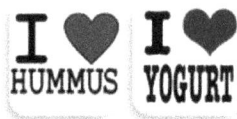

Greek Yogurt
Good: High in protein
Bad: Lactose (if lactose intolerant)

CHAPTER FOUR

Processed Foods

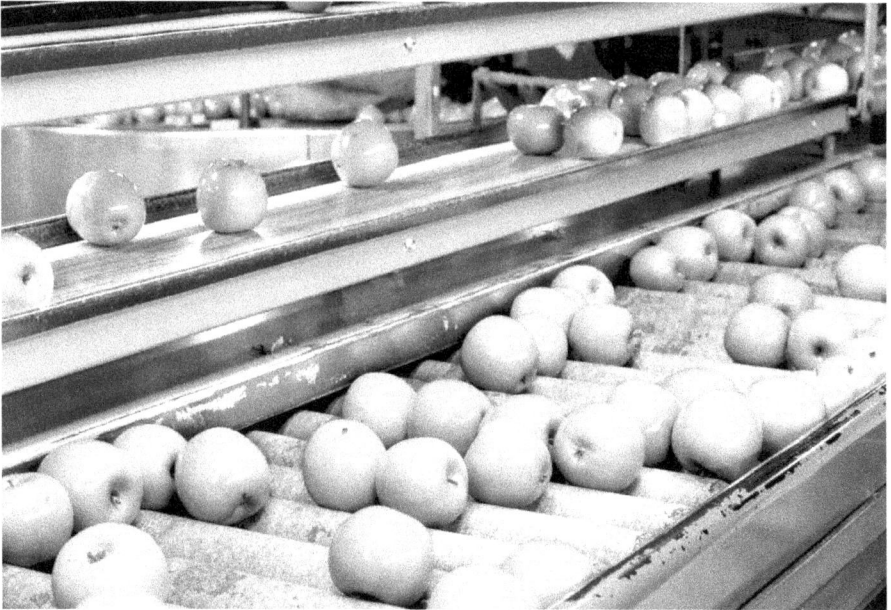

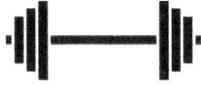

W hat comes to mind when you hear the phrase "processed foods"? What kinds of processes does that term refer to?

Many people think of processed foods as being bad for them or "not healthy", but what they don't realize is that every piece of food we consume—and every ingredient going into those foods—has gone through some sort of process to either make it safer for you to eat or to increase its functionality in baking or cooking.

Everything is processed!

Even something as simple as an apple has gone through a process of harvesting, washing, bagging, and storing prior to your purchase at the store (and eventual consumption at home or at work). Even more so, if those apples are chopped up and sold in the frozen aisle, they were not only harvested and cleaned, but also heat treated to prevent deterioration and break down, even in those freezing temperatures.

Let's go a step further and ask about flour. Processed? Not processed? Think about how flour exists in nature. There is no flour tree or flour pond. Cereal grains, whether it's wheat, rice, or corn, are used to create wheat flour, rice flour, and corn flour through a series of grinders and sieves, allowing the wheat kernels (or rice or corn) to be broken down and ground into smaller pieces, eventually becoming small enough to call it flour.

But before you can even begin to grind the kernels, the raw ingredient goes through similar processes as the raw apple did, including harvesting, cleaning, and sometimes drying of the wheat, rice, and corn.

Ok I get it. That's not what you mean by processed foods. You're talking about something like a frozen dinner that might contain prepared pasta, pre-cooked meat, with added flavors and seasonings. You don't like the fact that there are words on the back of the package that you can't understand.

While I can't make an umbrella statement about all packaged products and all ingredients, everything going into your food is still food:

1. The prepared pasta was cooked the same way you would have cooked it at home—just on a larger scale.

2. The cooked meat was cooked beforehand to make it easier for you (otherwise you wouldn't be able to make a 10-minute meal for your family).

3. Those flavors, seasonings, and other added ingredients are meant to make the food taste better (unless you want to eat some bland pasta) and meant to keep the product safe while you store it in your refrigerator or freezer.

No ingredient is added unnecessarily; there are always reasons for the ingredient, and just because it is a word you don't understand, doesn't mean it's completely foreign (more on this topic in the next chapter).

The term "processed foods" typically refers to something that isn't "natural" or "pure" and isn't converted away from its natural state to create something new. But this terminology can often be misleading.

Let's try this again—maybe something like milk. Milk is natural and pure, right? It comes straight from the cow and nothing is done to alter its form. Wrong.

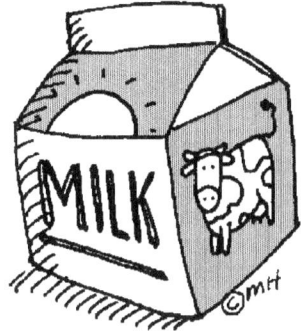

The majority of milk that is used and consumed in the U.S. is indeed processed in some way, depicted by the image below. Unless you live on a farm or go out of your way to buy raw milk (which I wouldn't advise), rarely will you ever drink non-processed milk.

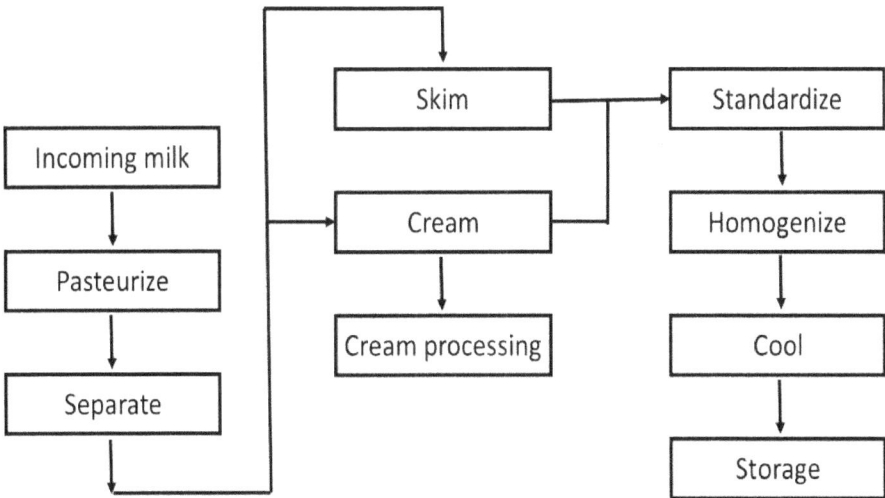

While milk is processed before you consume it, those processes are meant to make the milk safe for consumption and pleasantly delicious. These processes also have long and complex names, but don't be scared: **homogenization** helps break down the fat globules so you don't swallow big chunks of fat with your morning breakfast, **pasteurization** helps kill dangerous bacteria so that you do not get sick or die, **separation** and **standardization** helps ease the process of providing you with reduced fat and fat-free milk options.

Milk can be sold whole, with reduced fat, fat-free, or it can be used as an ingredient in other foods like cheese, butter, cookies, and sauces; now there's even a lactose-free high-protein version of cow's milk—and it's delicious by the way!

Whether you drink milk alone or other dairy products, you are consuming a processed food. Without the homogenization, pasteurization, and other processes shown in the diagram, the milk you know of today would look and taste completely different.

What do you think now... would you consider milk as a natural food or a processed food? Maybe both? The same way that a food being good and bad for you is not as straightforward as you would think, the idea of processing food goes far beyond the grocery store.

CHAPTER FIVE

Food Aisle Deceptions

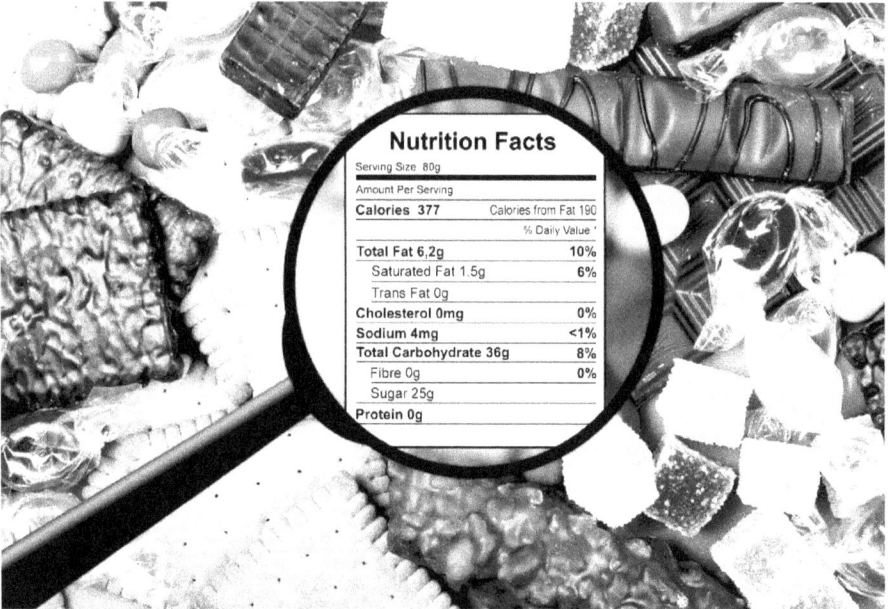

Nutrition Facts

Serving Size 80g

Amount Per Serving

Calories 377	Calories from Fat 190
	% Daily Value *
Total Fat 6,2g	10%
Saturated Fat 1.5g	6%
Trans Fat 0g	
Cholesterol 0mg	0%
Sodium 4mg	<1%
Total Carbohydrate 36g	8%
Fibre 0g	0%
Sugar 25g	
Protein 0g	

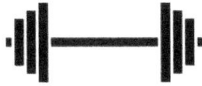

I've really grown to love the weekly (and sometimes daily) trips to the supermarket. To me it's like an adventure, picking which fruits to snack on that week and choosing which vegetables we will be roasting for our lunches.

The problem, though, is that once you start paying attention to the food you are consuming, and once you understand more about each individual ingredient and product, trips to the grocery store are never quick and easy.

Walking through the aisles, I might know that I want to buy tomato sauce, but then I have to sit and compare every option on the shelf. First I start by looking at the price. Then I see which jar is bigger than the other. Lastly, I turn the package around and compare nutrition labels and ingredient lines. *Why does this one cost an extra fifty cents? Which one has protein in it? Do they both have the same amount of sodium?*

All sorts of questions come to mind when looking at product packaging; not only can the back of the package be confusing with all the "chemically sounding" ingredients, but the front of the package can be just as unclear, trying to understand what it actually means to be "gluten free" and "made without steroids." While some of the front-of-pack call-outs can be helpful in selecting one product over another, even a food scientist can be overwhelmed by the excessive symbols and flags on food packages—which are designed to *encourage the sale* of the product, no matter how good, bad, sugary, or salty it is.

In this chapter, I hope to point out some of the phrases and words that are commonly misconstrued and attempt to explain their meanings. By having a better understanding of what these call-outs mean (if they mean anything at all), reading labels and packages can be that much easier. Thus, your trip to the grocery store can be more enjoyable as well.

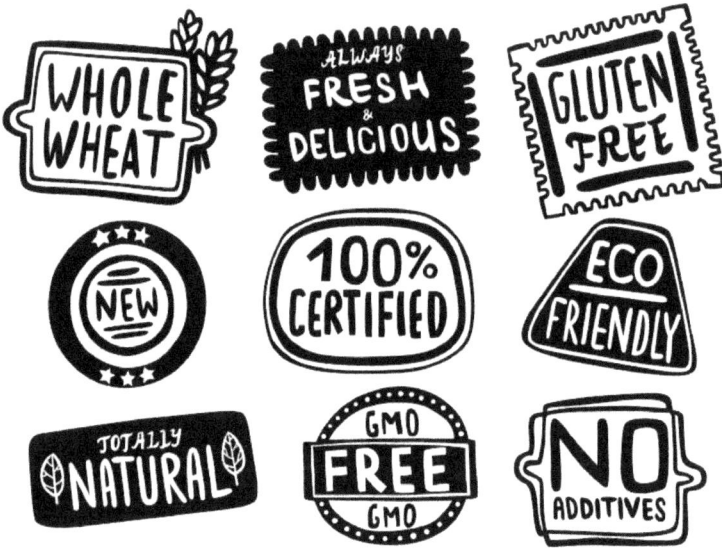

Call-outs on Packaging: Don't let them fool you!

The first thing you need to realize is that most words or phrases used on product packaging are strategically worded and placed to encourage consumer sales. There's probably a good reason why a snack bar is called *Wheat Bar* as opposed to just *Snack Bar*. There's probably a good reason why the front of the package reads "gluten free" or "contains organic oats."

The package is basically an advertisement!

In the first instance, the company who made the *Wheat Bar* wants you to know without a doubt that the snack bar contains wheat, so by putting the word in the name, there's no question (or is there?).

As for gluten free and organic, the product is targeted toward that particular audience; the company selling the product wants the organic and gluten-free community to know right off the bat that the product is an excellent choice for them—since it contains (or doesn't contain) key ingredients.

But just because something is called out on the package, that doesn't mean it's good. Just because the name of the product is *Wheat Bar* doesn't mean it is 100% whole wheat. In fact, it doesn't even mean it is *whole* wheat; all it really means is that some type of wheat is an ingredient in the bar. So in this case, the ingredient "enriched flour" is just as likely as "whole wheat flour."

What's the difference you might ask?

Wheat kernels are made up of three things: bran, endosperm, and germ (see image). For whole wheat, all three parts are intact. For white wheat, the bran and germ are removed, leaving the endosperm all by itself.

ANATOMY OF A GRAIN

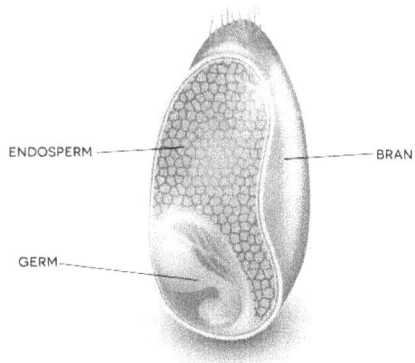

ENDOSPERM

BRAN

GERM

In the past years, consumers have been told to increase their intake of whole wheat products (as opposed to products from white flour) because it contains higher amounts of fiber. To some, whole wheat is considered healthier than white wheat flour because the entire piece of wheat kernel is used. White wheat is often called "enriched flour" because there are important vitamins and minerals contained in the bran and germ that are added back (or enriched) to the white flour in processing.

So when it comes down to it, both whole wheat flour and white flour are *wheat* flour. The company selling you that *Wheat Bar* is taking advantage of the fact that you as a consumer want to increase your whole wheat intake, while knowing that you most likely have no idea what the difference is between the two wheat flours. Don't be fooled! Look for some indication on the package that it is made from "100% whole wheat."

As for gluten-free and organic, there are rules that need to be followed in order to use these phrases on food packages. However, just because a product indicates gluten-free, doesn't mean it is any more special than alternatives that don't put those words on the package.

For example, corn does not contain gluten. EVER. Corn NEVER has gluten in it. So anything that is typically made from corn (instead of wheat or other gluten-containing grains) would be gluten-free. If you compare a regular box of corn tacos to a specially marked "gluten-free" box of corn tacos, you will most likely find that they are both gluten-free, just one decided to write the words on the front while the other opted out.

The "organic oats" call-out is a completely different topic, but, to put it simply, there still are debates whether organic is healthier for you than conventional foods. Also, when it comes to organic, "contains organic oats" indicates that the ingredient *oats* is organic, while that product most likely contains a handful of other ingredients that are not organic. If the oats are the only ingredient in the entire package that is organic (while the others are not organic) are the potential benefits of organic still viable?

No call-out? Don't worry.

In order to use some phrases and call-outs on packages, certain guidelines must be followed, and the company must retain documentation that the claim is in fact true. Though, in some instances there are phrases and call-outs that are *not required by law* to be labeled on a product; in other words—if you elect to claim it, you can, but if you don't want to claim it, you don't have to.

As already discussed, gluten-free is a great example. If your target consumer is not the gluten-free consumer, then you might choose to not indicate the gluten-free nature of your product on the package.

Similarly, if the package or serving size contains "only 100 calories", those words do not *need* to be called out on the front— but you can if you want. If you choose to use those words on the package, you must be prepared to show documentation that your recipe reflects your claim if needed (like in an audit or court proceedings).

Sometimes, it is not beneficial for a company to use a claim or a call-out, so they do not list it on the front of the package. Depending on the product and ingredients, reading the back and side labels can quickly alert you of some of these call-outs (if you know what you are looking for).

Overall, it is important to learn on your own to look past the call-outs on the package. Not only can they be confusing since all the company really wants to do is *sell its product,* sometimes the call-outs can be incorrect or illegally placed.

There are many examples of companies that have claimed something on their package and later penalized by the government for false labeling. While the penalty may be monetary and part of their punishment may be to change their packaging (consumers may never know), this does not prevent them from making the same mistake again. It also does not prevent **other** companies from making the same mistake.[6, 7] If the mistake is made again, the company at fault would just be punished again. In some cases, if the company reaps enough benefits in terms of sales and brand exposure, and is prepared for the repercussions, the false labeling might be worth it.

However, no matter the size of the company, labeling mistakes can be costly. Not only are there hefty fines from the government and legal costs, but also expenses associated with printing new packages and the liability in any falsely labeled packaging that would need to be thrown away.[8]

Not all companies follow the rules!

A few years ago, the FDA found evidence that Castle Cheese, Inc. had been labeling their Parmesan and romano cheese products incorrectly. Documentation from the FDA stated that their "product labels declare that the products are Parmesan cheese or romano cheese, but they are in fact a mixture of trimmings of various cheeses and other ingredients" indicating that the product being labeled as Parmesan cheese may not have been 100% Parmesan. This labeling issue eventually led the company to bankruptcy.[5]

There are plenty other examples of unclear, unsubstantiated, or simply untrue claims being used by companies to market their products. In a report by the Center for Science in the Public Interest, one concerning case dealing with children's breakfast cereal is detailed as follows:

"In the fall of 2009, Kellogg's Cocoa Krispies proclaimed that it 'now helps support your child's immunity' (a concern of many parents during flu season), because it is fortified with vitamins A, B, C, and E. While a severe deficiency in those vitamins could interfere with the proper functioning of the body's immune system (and any other system), there is no evidence that Cocoa Krispies actually improves children's immune status or wards off disease. Moreover, the cereal is almost 40% sugar, containing 12 g per ¾ cup (31 g) serving."[7]

In other words, the company was claiming that the breakfast cereal helped boost children's immune systems. However, no direct evidence shows that *the cereal itself* was actually beneficial in boosting immune health. While the company may not be intentionally deceiving the customer, it's all a matter of wording and opinion. ***All the more reason to understand what's in your food and on the label!***

Some food companies are much more conservative and trust-worthy than others when it comes to choosing a proper name for a food product and providing information on packaging (to not false advertise or mislead the consumer into buying the product). Not all companies try to deceive you, but it can be hard to discern between the good guys and bad guys.

Whole Wheat

For me, the hardest thing is to walk into the bread aisle and choose a bread that is good for me. Aside from the question of "What does good for me really mean?" the bread aisle is filled with white bread, whole wheat, honey wheat, wheat, and multi-grain varieties that can easily frustrate a shopper.

Truthfully, you need to answer the "good for me" question before deciding on a bread. Do you want a bread that's good for you in terms of high fiber? Or do you want a bread that's good for you in terms of macros?

As described before, if you're looking for more fiber, whole wheat is the way to go—but you need to read that label and make sure it is 100% whole wheat (if it's just called *wheat*, it might not be 100%). If you're not concerned with fiber and all you want is the carbohydrates, proteins, and fat, choose any type of bread. Most breads have comparable amounts of macros, seeing as they add sugar and fat for flavor and texture (the same thing that you would do if you made bread at home). All varieties contain essential vitamins and minerals, although white breads are enriched while the whole wheats may or may not be enriched or fortified.

Protein Powder

Not all protein powders are created equal. While specialty stores and vitamin shops are where you will find the most options of protein powders including egg, plant, whey, and beef proteins, you can still buy whey protein at many grocery stores instead of making a separate trip to the vitamin shop. I don't like to buy my protein powder at the grocery store because they are usually not in the purest form.

The purest form of protein powder would be protein and protein only. This would mean the powder is unflavored and does not contain added sweeteners—flavors and sweeteners both enhance flavor and affect overall taste.

Most of the proteins that I have found in grocery stores contain sugars, artificial sweeteners, and other additives that are meant to make the powder taste better; I always prefer the pure simplest protein powder, and I will add my own flavors and sugar to my protein shake, if desired.

Whey protein is the most commonly discussed type of protein powder. It is a by-product of the cheese-making process, meaning it is left over after cheese is made; further purification and water removal from this ingredient leads to the dry powder form we are all used to. The purest form of whey protein commercially available is whey protein isolate (WPI) and is typically found in products that contain the term "ISO" in the name. Just look for the words "Whey Protein Isolates" on the label. If they are not isolates, they are still proteins, but may also contain other dairy components such as lactose and vitamins and minerals. Even some isolates have added ingredients—especially flavorings—so just read the label and make sure to get unflavored (if you can stomach it) or a flavor of your liking, but try to stay away from added sugars in your protein powder! In this case, the fewer the ingredients in the protein powder the better (and more pure).

Other protein powders come from their respective sources: egg, plant, beef, etc. Some proteins are better suited for baking, while others are best for drinking. If all you are looking for is a protein powder and you are not picky about certain characteristics, then choose your source based on taste and other personal preferences (if you're vegan definitely don't buy the whey!).

Weight Loss Foods

Diet beverages, fat-free products, and low calorie sweets are all examples of foods that could be aimed at folks who are trying to lose weight. Be wary when purchasing products that are specifically labeled as weight loss foods, though. Depending on the reasoning behind the categorization as such, it may not be any different than other products that are not specifically labeled for weight loss.

As was mentioned earlier, if a product is "healthy" but the company does not see added benefit in calling out to the consumer that it is healthy for whatever reason, then those benefits are hidden within the ingredient label on the back or side panel. For example, we all know that vegetables are good for you and full of vitamins and minerals, but how many times have you seen a package of lettuce shout out "EAT ME TO LOSE WEIGHT!"?

While some products may actually be beneficial for you when in weight loss mode, oftentimes people eat more than the suggested serving size of these foods, defeating the purpose of it. Meal replacement shakes and bars are a great example—they are called MEAL REPLACEMENTS for a reason. If you drink a shake or a bar for lunch, make sure you don't eat your regular lunch of pizza and fries as well (save that for dinner if you really have to!).

Also, be careful with weight loss foods because they can sometimes make you lazy without you even realizing; it may be easy to forgo exercising for the day or to snack on other foods because you think it's "ok" since you are eating this healthy weight loss food. So make sure not to make excuses when choosing these weight loss products.

Reduced Fat and Fat Free

When you remove one ingredient, you have to replace it with something else. In the case of reduced fat and fat-free products, it could be water, sugar, or other carbohydrates. Read the label before purchasing because you might be surprised to find out that reduced fat does not mean reduced calories.

I experienced a huge disappointment once when reaching for reduced fat peanut butter instead of regular peanut butter. I *love* peanut butter! But I was trying to be more calorie-conscience, so I chose the healthier version—or so I thought. Come to find out, the particular reduced fat peanut butter that I purchased indeed contained fewer grams of fat than its regular counterpart, but the grams of fat were replaced with grams of carbohydrates. In the end, both products contained the same amount of calories, so it did not benefit me at all (I was counting macros at the time, and the fat was actually needed more than the carbohydrates).

One thing to remember with fat is that just because a product is labeled "fat-free" doesn't mean it's anything special. I've seen gummy candies with that call-out before; in case you didn't know, a basic gummy candy recipe is just water, sugar, and gelatin—never a pinch of fat in sight.

Sugar-free and Artificial Sweeteners

In the case of sweeteners, when you remove sucrose (everyday table sugar) from a product, if you are trying to make a similar product with similar sweetness intensity, you have to replace it something as well. That something can be *artificial sweeteners* like aspartame, sucralose, or acesulfame potassium or *natural sweeteners* like stevia. While the sweetness of these sugar replacers come somewhat close to the sweetness level of sugar, they carry a bitter note with them to which some people are sensitive.

Labeling of these ingredients can be misleading at times. Personally, I do not like the taste of any sweeteners that are not sugar. For instance, if a label indicates "no artificial sweeteners" I get excited and grab for the package. With further investigation, I then find that what they meant was they use stevia instead of aspartame or sucralose. They weren't trying to tell me that they use sugar (or no sweeteners at all), but that the sweeteners are not artificial. Stevia is not considered an artificial sweetener because it comes from a natural plant source, hence the natural classification. Nonetheless, this natural source is not any better than the artificial source, since I don't like the bitter aftertaste of either of them.

If you don't mind the taste of sugar replacers, then by all means, drink them! Eat them! Just be careful not to overconsume. Some studies have shown that these sweeteners actually assist in weight gain rather than weight loss, for multiple reasons.[9, 10] Yet, if you're like me and can't stand the taste of these replacers, read the label carefully before buying!

Furthermore, potential side effects of overconsumption include cancer and other health hazards;[9, 10] for example, while sugar alcohols—like maltitol and erythritol—may be beneficial in achieving the same sweetness level of sugar, diabetics have reported having a negative response to them the same way they have a negative response to sugar.[11, 12] Just as with all other foods, with the good must also come the bad.

Chemicals and Preservatives

Some companies like to label on their packages "No Preservatives" or "Contains No Chemicals." As a smart consumer, you should look beyond the call-out and think about the words that are being used: preservatives and chemicals.

What is a preservative? It is an ingredient that is used to *preserve* a food, or help it last longer (increase its shelf life).

What is a chemical? It is an ingredient that has constant chemical composition and that is composed of elements on the periodic table.

Salt is both those things. Common table salt. NaCl. Sodium chloride. Salting is one of the oldest forms of preserving foods such as bacon, pickles, and salted fish. While the words preservative and chemical can sound scary, understand that salt is an example of both of these things, and then you should recognize that those words aren't always bad things.

There are other preservatives and chemicals with names that seem unrecognizable on ingredient labels (*e.g.* acetic acid and ascorbic acid), but do your research on the meanings and the compositions of those hard-to-pronounce words before jumping to conclusions. There are plenty of hard-to-pronounce words that are perfectly natural and come straight from Mother Nature; don't let words scare you! (Acetic acid is in vinegar and ascorbic acid in lemon juice.)

And remember, preservatives are added to a food to ensure it is safe to eat by the time it gets to you—and if you don't eat it immediately, you can keep it in your cupboard or refrigerator for a few days. If you don't want so many of these things in your foods, the best option is to bring back the cookie jar #CookieJar and start making your own foods at home!

Natural, Organic, and Gluten Free

These three topics are very controversial, but also are very important topics, so I will touch on them briefly. My intention in explaining a little bit about these things is to inform, not to force my opinion on you... so here, let's take a stab at it.

Natural. To this day, this word has **no concrete definition** in the United States when it comes to food. On the contrary, organic and gluten free are clearly defined and have regulations surrounding the use of these terms on any product labels. The word natural can be loosely used to describe foods that come "naturally" from the earth or contain "natural" ingredients. Next time you look at a food and it deems itself "natural" don't let this marketing tactic sway you to purchase one item over another. Assumptions can be made about what that call-out means, but there is no standard to define and monitor the use of this word—yet.

Since the meaning of "natural" is slightly ambiguous, it can be seen on labels of many types of products. Back in 2006, Cadbury Schweppes reformulated their 7UP soft drink, resulting in new packaging using the claim "Now 100% Natural" and the claim "stripped of the artificial stuff" in advertisements. After a few months, the company decided to remove the natural call-out from the label, due to complaints and lawsuit filings that deemed the term misleading to consumers. This is just one example of the questionable use of the natural claim, but since not all products receive attention at the same level of 7UP, it is possible that other claims could remain on packaging for years without complaints. Be cautious when purchasing your next snack based on the thought that it is a "natural" food product.

Organic. Another thing to pay attention to is any organic food that you are eating. While organic does have a definition that is regulated in the United States, there are differences between "100% organic" products and foods that "contain organic ingredients." Be cautious since some foods can contain both organic and non-organic ingredients; if they meet certain criteria, the product can be labeled as "contains organic [ingredient]" even when the remaining ingredients are not organic. Know what you're buying, and if you want something that is completely organic, look for the certified USDA organic seal or a "100% organic" claim that is reserved for products entirely composed of certified organic materials.

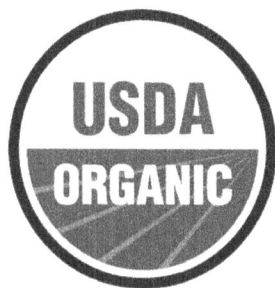

Gluten free. Gluten is a protein. It is not an alien, nor is it any type of foreign matter that is added to foods. Whatever other explanations you may have heard about where gluten comes from—forget about them! Gluten is a protein that is naturally found in wheat and other grains (like barley and rye). Any food that contains wheat will henceforth contain gluten too. There are plenty of foods that do not—NEVER have and NEVER will—contain gluten, such as potatoes, tapioca, beans, corn, and rice.

It's important to know what foods do and do not have gluten because there are some people that are sensitive to gluten to the point that ingestion of it can cause adverse effects like vomiting and joint pain. Gluten only adversely affects a person who has a clinical *sensitivity* or *intolerance* to gluten; similarly, if a food is gluten-free that doesn't automatically make it any more nutritious or contributory to weight loss than a similar product that does contain gluten.

Fortified and Enriched

When you read the next chapter about *macro*nutrients, realize that there are also things called *micro*nutrients. The micronutrients category includes vitamins and minerals, all of which are essential to proper body function. Some vitamins and minerals are sensitive to food processing practices like heat and light, but to make up for what was lost, the vitamins are added back in. In other words, a food that might naturally have high levels of a vitamin might lose some vitamins during processing, but synthetic vitamins would be added so the level goes back to the original high level of vitamin.

The process of adding vitamins to foods is fortification. Any food that is fortified has had additional micronutrients added to it for any number of reasons. One reason could be that vitamins were lost during processing—this is more commonly known as *enrichment*. For example, iron and B vitamins (naturally found in wheat) can be lost during milling and grinding of wheat into flour. These vitamins and minerals are then enriched back into the flour to replenish what was lost, hence the existence of these micronutrients on flour and bread labels (*e.g.* folic acid, niacin).

Another reason for fortification could be that the food doesn't naturally contain that vitamin. To ensure we consume enough of the vitamin in our diets (and do not become deficient), those micronutrients are fortified into a food for our benefit. So if a cookie is fortified with vitamins or if a sports drink is fortified with minerals, those micronutrients may not have been there originally, but they are meant to provide some added benefit to the consumer.

Fortification in most cases is good because then we can consume most of our essential vitamins and minerals through our diet, as opposed to taking supplemental pills. However, make sure you are not misled by foods that use fortification as a marketing ploy. Most people would consider it unnecessary to have fortified gummy bears or candy bars—but if you don't get your micronutrients from anywhere else, then maybe it's beneficial for you (just maybe)!

Soy Alternatives

Soy alternatives have been popping up left and right on the market over the last few years. As I've stated a few times already about other types of alternatives, these are not necessarily better for you than the product that the alternative was designed to replace.

Some examples of soy alternatives are soy milk, soy cheese, and tofu. Soy is one of eight of the nation's major food allergens, so for some people it is essential that they do not consume any of these soy products. However, there are people that are allergic to dairy and are lactose intolerant, so they cannot consume cow's milk and other cow's milk products like cheese and yogurt—in this case, soy is a practical option.

Meanwhile, there are other people that are vegan or vegetarian or simply choose not to consume these dairy products. For those who have a specific reason to not eat a food, an alternative exists. This gives people options; a vegetarian can still celebrate Thanksgiving, they just might eat a tofu turkey instead of a real turkey.

Similar to gluten-free products, these soy products do not necessarily provide additional benefits to people who do not *dietarily* need to choose soy products. Quite contrarily, there have been studies that show a potential connection between soy consumption and hormone disruption, although it is not a definitive link between the two.[13, 14, 15]

In the end, my message to you is simple. Read beyond the package and beyond the label. Realize that food companies are just trying to sell to you. Colors on the package, words and call-outs, as well as special ingredients are not used by mistake. While most companies take time to ensure their labeling is not misleading or deceitful, there are companies out there that may not be as conservative. Be a smart consumer, and think about what you buy before you buy it!

CHAPTER SIX

Count Your Macros

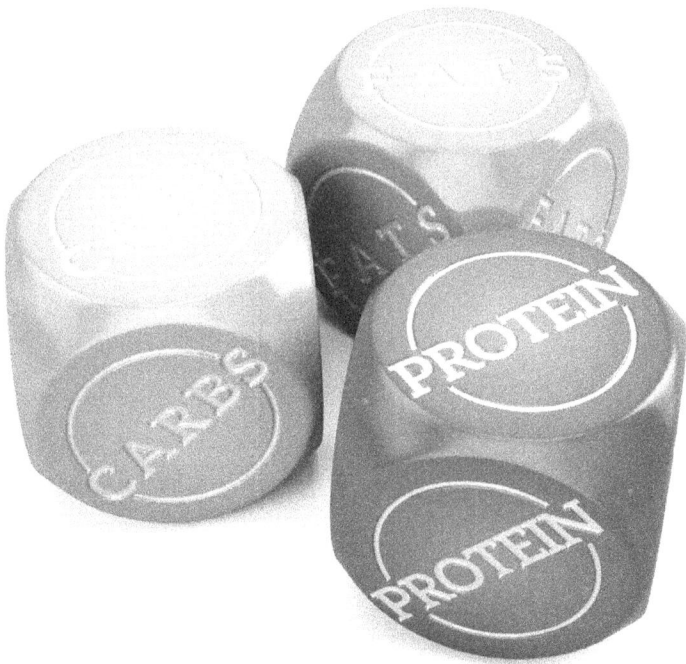

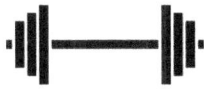

M acros. This year's buzzword. Every fit person on social media talks about "counting macros", "hitting their macros", and "if it fits your macros" (#IIFYM). Hopefully you caught it, but even I have mentioned the term macros a few times in this book already.

Macros is simply a shorthand term for the longer and not-so-hard-to-say word *macronutrients*. In nutrition and food science, when we talk about macronutrients, we are referring to those essential nutrients that provide our bodies with *calories* or *energy*.

Calorie is a measure of the amount of energy that would be provided to the human body as it burns and utilizes the macronutrient. The more calories we consume, the more units we have to go toward our daily energy expenditure.

However, any energy that is not used, is stored as fat for future use (just in case!). So if you eat 2000 calories and sit on the couch all day, you don't expend a lot of energy and many of those 2000 calories are stored for later; on the other hand, if you eat 2000 calories and run a marathon, you will expend a lot of energy and most of those calories will be used to give you energy to run rather than stored as fat as you sit and watch your favorite television show.

More specifically, *carbohydrates*, *protein*, and *fat* are the macronutrients that provide our bodies with energy. Carbohydrates and protein provide our bodies with 4 calories per gram, while fats provide more than double that (9 calories per gram). Scientists may also include water and alcohol as macronutrients: water since it is essential to the body, even though it provides zero calories, and alcohol since it provides calories, although it is not essential to the body.

To start, the only thing essential to know about alcohol is that it does in fact provide calories to your body (7 calories per gram of alcohol). Ever wonder why some people lose weight as soon as they graduate from college and move back home? Or did you ever wonder why you have a tough time losing weight when you go drinking every weekend even though your diet is on point all week? While it is easy to mentally ignore the calories provided by alcohol, it is just as easy to physically replace that alcohol with a glass of drinking water.

Drink more water!

Water is in fact essential for the body to survive—after all, our bodies are composed of approximately 65% water! Ever wonder why gym rats carry around a gallon of water with them as they work out? They might even have the gallon with them at work or at home. I cannot overstress the importance of water; not only can water reduce feelings of hunger, but drinking more water has been shown to make you look younger by reducing puffiness and blemishes in the face, among other things.[16]

Next time you feel hungry, try drinking a glass of water before you grab for a candy bar; that feeling may in fact be thirst instead of hunger. Yes, drinking more water will increase your trips to the bathroom, but that's nothing new to all the fit people you follow on Instagram.

Alcohol and water are not the macros that everyone focuses on; for that, we have to discuss carbohydrates, proteins, and fat. Every food you consume is made up of a combination of fat, carbohydrates, and protein, as illustrated below. The green, yellow, and blue guys (dark grey, light grey, and grey) are the macronutrients that make up each food, in this instance, bread.

Some foods can contain copious amounts of a single macro, like celery and bananas, which have minimal fat and protein, but lots of carbohydrates (lots of yellow/light grey guys!). Other foods, like avocadoes, have a generous mix of all three macros (a good mix of all three guys!).

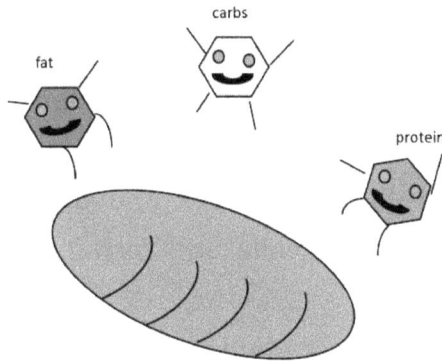

What Are Macros?

What really are macros though? What do they do for you? Why is everyone so concerned with macros?

Macronutrients are in fact molecules—chemicals if you will—that consist of carbon, hydrogen, and oxygen (and nitrogen in protein). These macronutrients are building blocks of the food we eat; the food we eat is a combination of carbs, protein, and fat.

Let's compare the macronutrient concept to jewelry; think about a 10K gold necklace. While the final product is molded

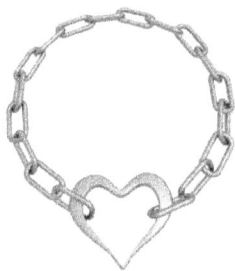

into a specific shape, the necklace itself is a composite of gold, copper, and other metals. Those metals are on the same level as macronutrients. They are small building blocks that make up the final product; carbohydrates, proteins, and fats (the metals in this example) are composited together in specific ratios to make up and form each of the foods that we eat (the necklace).

Macro Diet

The macro diet is the basis behind the Junk Food Fit program. By understanding what our food is made of, we can calculate not only **calories** for total energy, but also the individual **macros** themselves to control how our energy is used. It is the reason that the Junk Food Fit program allows you to eat cupcakes, pizza, chocolate, and other "junk foods" (in moderation of course) while still losing weight and gaining muscle.

The theory behind counting macros is that a carb is a carb, a protein is a protein, and fat is fat, no matter what source you get it from (in terms of energy). So if a bowl of rice and chicken has 40 grams of carbohydrates, 30 grams of protein, and 10 grams of fat, you can in theory eat a snack bar with the same 40:30:10 macro breakdown instead.

In simple terms, you are going to be adding up the amount of green guys, yellow guys, and blue guys in your diet. If you are supposed to eat 50 yellow guys in one day, you can get those yellow guys from any food you wish—just keep track and don't go over 50! With this concept, it doesn't matter whether you eat completely clean and have meals of chicken, rice, and broccoli, or if you eat "dirty" and have a slice of pizza here and there (as long as you don't go over your limits).

Of course this concept doesn't take into consideration internal healthfulness (*e.g.* saturated fats being bad for you while unsaturated fats are better for your overall health), but it has nonetheless proven time and time again to help people lose weight. I myself swear by this method, as it has been the only method that has allowed me to stay fit while eating cookies at my job every day—and the only effective method used to finally dip my weight below 140 pounds (I haven't been that light since high school!).

Counting macros takes time and dedication in that you must remember to record everything that you eat and keep track. But over time it becomes easier; over time you begin to understand what macros are in each food without even calculating it or entering into a counting macros app on your phone.

That's the goal: to learn how to make better choices. I don't want you living the rest of your life counting calories and macros day in and day out. What I want is for you to use counting macros as a method to teach yourself about the food, to understand what you are putting into your body, and to empower yourself to live a better and healthier life.

In the next few chapters, you will learn a little bit about each of these individual macros, and more on how to track what you eat. Also, a more detailed description of the Macro Diet can be found in Chapter 10.

CHAPTER SEVEN

Carbohydrates

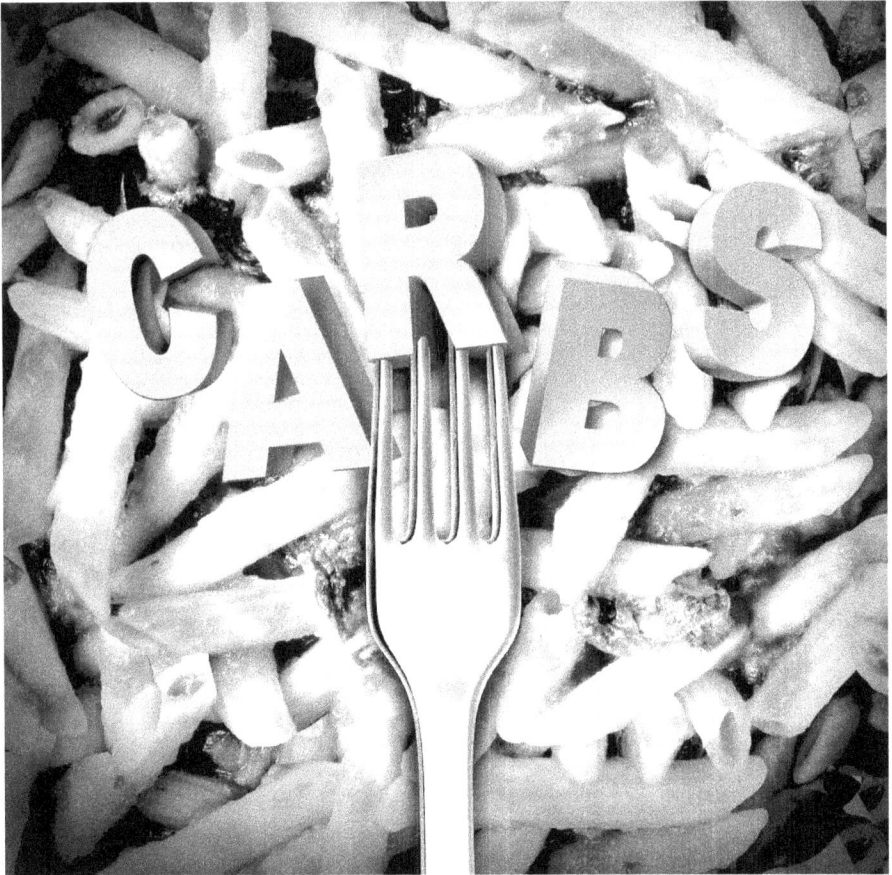

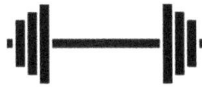

Foods like bread, pasta, rice, and potatoes are not carbohydrates in themselves, but they are excellent *sources* of carbs. Those foods are like the 10K gold necklace, while the carbs are the gold that makes the necklace.

Try not to get confused though, carbs in each food come in different types, ranging from sugar to starch to fiber. Sugar, starch, and fiber are all carbohydrates even though they may taste differently and provide various types of energy to an individual.

Simply put, sugar (glucose) is used by your body in order to keep it running properly. The same way you add gas to your car to make it work, your body needs sufficient sugar per day to keep it working at full power.

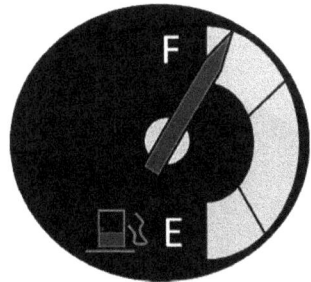

Your carb gas tank

Your body, of course, can break down larger carbohydrates like starch in order to make the sugar it needs (this is not an excuse for you to eat candy all day). Even the sugars in candy are broken down to a smaller sugar that is more easily utilized by the body (sucrose and glucose are both sugars, but different from each other!).

Without going too deep into it, sugar provides "instant" energy while starch takes longer to break down and metabolize, often referred to as "sustained" energy. Fiber is similar to starch, but it is much harder for our body to digest, so it isn't known for providing energy but instead for its digestive tract cleansing capabilities.

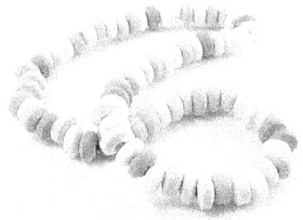

Let's go back to the jewelry analogy. This time instead of picturing a gold necklace, imagine one of those candy necklaces. Each piece of candy is like sugar, the smallest building block of carbohydrates. By adding more candies to the chain, you are building longer chains of carbs, similar to starches. And the harder it is for you to bite off a piece of the candy from the chain, the closest it is to being a fiber or indigestible starch. Sugars, starches, and fibers are all carbohydrates, they just have different characteristics (yellow vs. pink vs. orange candy pieces) and contribute differently to the overall candy necklace.

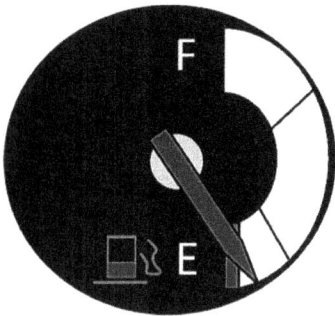

While sugars and longer chained carbs are necessary for survival, the human body also has the ability to convert fat and protein into sugars, in the case when your carb gas tank is on E.

When counting macros, you must keep the gas tank in mind. You need to consume enough carbs each day to keep your body functioning properly. The moment your body runs out of gas and there is no more food to work with, it will start utilizing the energy that your body has put on reserve, first using glycogen (storage carbohydrates) then moving on to body fat and protein in muscles.

Gas tank at empty

This is why it is so important to make sure you don't eat TOO FEW calories. Once your body doesn't receive calories from food, it finds another way to get energy—sometimes going into disaster mode and *storing* fat instead of *using* fat (the body is trying to take care of itself, and for all it knows, it's starving and may not have food for days on end).

The percent of each macro you consume per day should also take into account the gas tank concept. In deciding your macro breakdown (40% carbs, 30% protein, 30% fat or whatever your percentages might be), remember that you NEED a certain amount of carbs for the gas tank. Then, in order to build muscle, you NEED a certain amount of protein, and lastly, in order to absorb fat-soluble vitamins and keep your bodily processes functioning properly, you NEED a certain amount of fat. Each number of "need" varies from person to person, but you should never just cut one macro out completely or else your body will suffer in one way or another.

CHAPTER EIGHT

Protein

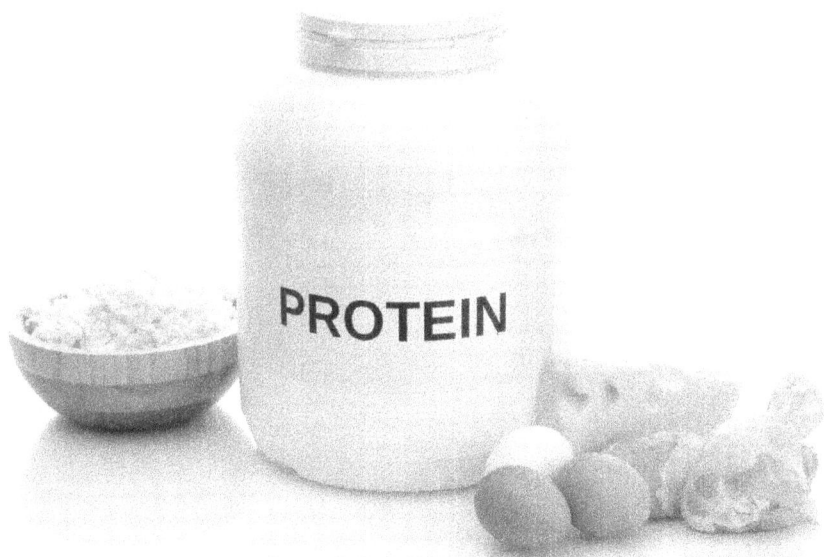

P roteins are similar to carbs in that they are also chains of smaller building block pieces. Instead of being a "necklace" made up of *sugars*, proteins are chains—or necklaces—made up of *amino acids* (AA). There are multiple kinds of amino acids, and every protein is made up of a combination of those different amino acids in chain form, both essential and non-essential (as shown to the right).

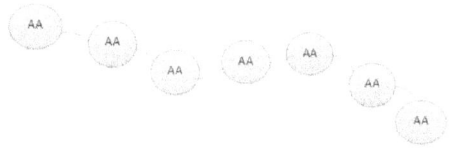

While the terms "essential" and "non-essential" may lead you to believe that some AAs are more important than others, that is not entirely true. The main difference is that the essential AAs must be consumed through food and your diet. The non-essential amino acids can be produced by your body and do not need to be directly supplied through food. There are nine total amino acids that are essential and eleven that are non-essential (see table).

Notice that these words may appear to be those so-called nasty "chemicals" in your food, but they are important in order to keep your body functioning properly. In some cases, they might be added to foods or

Essentials	Non-Essentials
Histidine	Arginine
Isoleucine	Cysteine
Leucine	Glycine
Lysine	Glutamine
Methionine	Proline
Phenylalanine	Tyrosine
Threonine	Alanine
Tryptophan	Aspartic Acid
Valine	Asparagine
	Glutamic Acid
	Serine

supplements, so make sure not to be scared by the "hard to pronounce" amino acids that you might spot on the label.

Contrary to belief, though, you don't have to eat meat to get your required daily intake of protein (although it is a lot easier if you do). Foods like beans and nuts are a good source of protein, but beans also are high in carbohydrates while nuts are high in fat. If you are looking for a great protein source with very few carbs and low percentages of fat, consider white meats like chicken and turkey. Fish is also a good source, but depending on the type of fish, it may be high in fat.

When at the grocery store, the trick is to look at the percent fat (%) labeled on the pack of meat. A meat labeled 85/15 has 15% fat while 93/7 only has 7% fat. Most ground meats have the fat % labeled, while steaks and cuts will not. The lower the fat, the less the flavor, yes, but the more protein and the healthier for you (in terms of fat consumption). If you need the fat, you can always add it yourself while cooking with butter or olive oil.

Another go-to source of protein is whole eggs. These are jam packed with all sorts of nutrients, considering their primary reason for being is to feed a growing chick (but don't worry, the eggs you buy at the store don't have baby chicks in them!). The whole egg will provide you protein, fat, some carbohydrates, as well as vitamins and minerals, while the egg white alone will provide you with all those things minus the fat and cholesterol.

You need protein to build muscle!

Having enough protein in your diet is most important when you are lifting weights and trying to build muscle. Think about it—when focusing on consuming enough protein in a day, what kinds of meat do you choose? You eat a turkey **leg**, chicken **thigh**, chicken **breast**, beef **shoulder**. They are all *muscles* from the animal. You eat animal muscles because they are high in protein.

Similarly, the human body's greatest content of protein is found in the muscles. Hence, you must consume protein to feed the growth of those muscles.

Besides muscle development, proteins are also essential for everyday processes that happen in your body. Proteins not only are used in building your muscles but are also key components of important enzymes, antibodies, and hormones—all necessary for proper functioning of your body.

Simply put, the protein that you consume goes first to those processes needed to keep your body functioning. Once all those processes are stable and sufficient, any extra protein can be used for muscle building. Because of this, oftentimes bodybuilders and fitness enthusiasts will consume supplemental amino acids and proteins in addition to the protein they get from food (commonly referred to as either "BCAAs" or "aminos"). This ensures that all the necessary bodily processes are taken care of, and then whatever food they eat, the protein can go straight to building muscle and to the body getting stronger.

Protein comes from many different types of foods, but nonetheless it can be difficult to find anything besides eggs and meat that contain high levels of protein; it is much easier to find foods full of carbohydrates and fat (especially junk foods) than with high amounts of proteins.

More recently, the food industry has noticed this gap in macro dieting, and more products on the grocery shelves are seen with "source of protein" call-out on the label. Just be careful when choosing these specifically for the high protein levels—sometimes the carb and fat levels are so high that it doesn't benefit you to consume as a protein source.

No matter the food source, individual proteins vary due to the types of amino acids that build them; at the same time, all protein provides the same 4 calories of energy per gram of protein eaten. Choose the type of protein that is best for you. After all, it is your journey and no one else's!

CHAPTER NINE

Fat

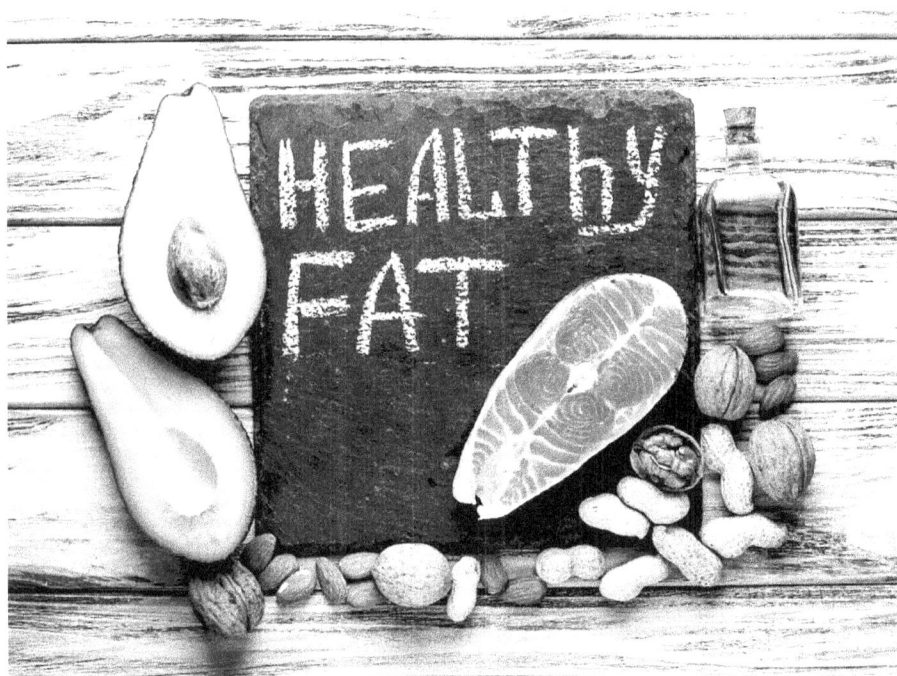

L eaving the best for last, let's now talk about fat as a macronutrient. Why is it the best? Merely because we all LOVE to eat fatty foods. Donuts, cakes, candy bars, pizza, fried chicken. The list goes on. Fat adds flavor after all, so why wouldn't we LOVE to eat fatty foods?

Fats are a bit complicated in that typical fat sources like olive oil and butter are not just one solid block of fat. They are made up of different fatty acids that can either be "good for you" like unsaturated fats or "bad for you" like saturated fats. The difference in the two is solely the amount of hydrogens covering the "necklace" of carbons, as depicted in the images to the right.

Unsaturated fats can come in two forms: monounsaturated and polyunsaturated. If you've ever looked at the nutrition facts panel of common foods, you'll notice both these words

TYPES & SOURCES of FATTY ACIDS

Unsaturated fats

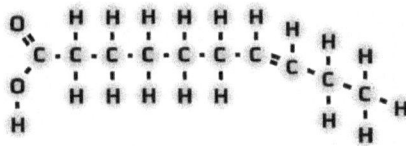

Satured fats

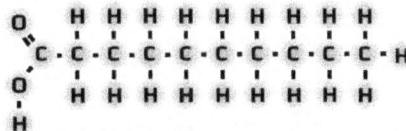

on the side. The difference has to do with the amount of hydrogens missing from the chain; *mono* merely means there is only one double bond, so two hydrogens are missing; *poly* means there is more than one double bond on the chain, so more than two hydrogens are missing. Omega-6 and Omega-3 fatty acids are types of polyunsaturateds.

Combinations of these polyunsaturated, monounsaturated, or saturated fatty acids make up the different kinds of fat sources. Depending on the fatty acid makeup of the fat source, this will make it "good for you" or "bad for you."

The following chart depicts the breakdown of certain fat sources by the fatty acid composition. Generally, higher amounts of saturated fats are found in fats from animals (like butter), while higher amounts of unsaturated fats are usually in plant oils (olive, canola). There are some that don't follow the rule, like coconut oil, which is sourced from a plant, but is high in saturated fats.

Compositions of Dietary Fats and Oils

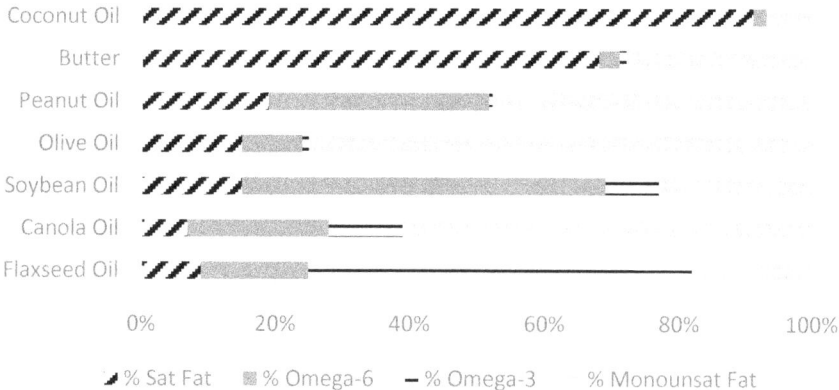

Legend: ◢ % Sat Fat   ▧ % Omega-6   — % Omega-3   % Monounsat Fat

Typically, a fat source is considered "good for you" when it has low levels of saturated fats and high levels of mono and poly unsaturated fatty acids. In terms of energy, no matter the type of fat, they all provide you with the same 9 calories per gram, but in terms of your internal health (heart disease, cholesterol), that's where saturated versus unsaturated makes a difference.

Unsaturated fats are generally recognized as being healthy: monounsaturated fats are considered healthy because they may improve blood cholesterol levels in your body;[17] polyunsaturateds are considered good for you (including omega-3 fats and omega-6 fats) partly because they are essential for bodily processes like hormone production.[17]

On the other hand, saturated fats are bad for you because they have been found to increase blood cholesterol and increase risk for heart disease.[17] Animal products are easy sources of saturated fats, while some plant products, like coconut oil, also contain high levels of these types of "bad" fats.

While the simplest way to intake fat for the day would be to drink a tablespoon of olive oil, that may not be the most practical method. The foods we eat on a regular basis contain mixtures of the different fat sources, sometimes even containing both animal and plant sources (*e.g.* butter and vegetable oil); it's not really a question of how or where you will get your fat from (plenty of foods have plenty of fat) it's more of a question of how will you control that intake—since it is *so easy* to find foods high in fat.

Overall, just watch your intake of fat, especially if your family history shows vulnerabilities to heart disease. Don't forget that a little yummy (yet fatty) treat here and there can be good for the soul, so you don't have to eliminate *every* piece of fatty food from your diet! Especially if you join the Junk Food Fit movement, counting macros will allow you room to enjoy those little treats throughout the week.

Bodies are Amazing!

Your body is an amazing machine!!!!

Our bodies are so amazing that when we don't consume enough food, it can survive off our fat reserves for a while. And if we don't consume enough of one macronutrient, it can use the others to replenish itself—to a certain extent.

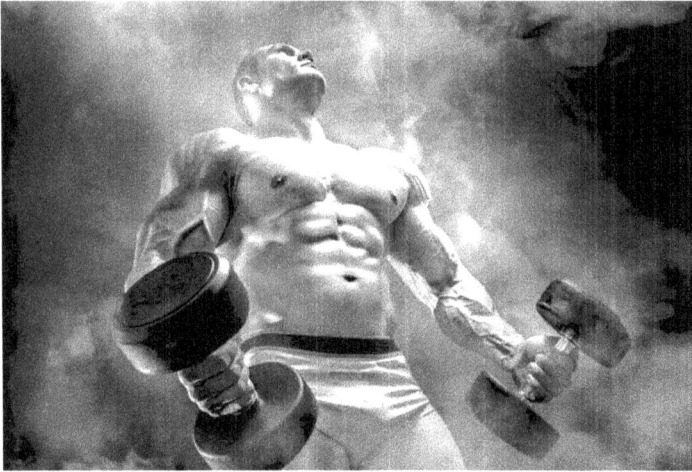

No matter the type of macronutrient, **any** excess is stored as fat, whether of carbs, protein, or fat, no matter if it's good or bad. Why is it stored? Just in case. The body is thinking ahead. *What if you can't afford to fill the gas tank tomorrow?* It knows then, it can use the fat stored in its reserve as energy to keep going.

Your body is amazing, and YOU are amazing. You have the strength, knowledge, and willpower to take weight by the horns and lose it! Keep reading to learn more.

meal Prep

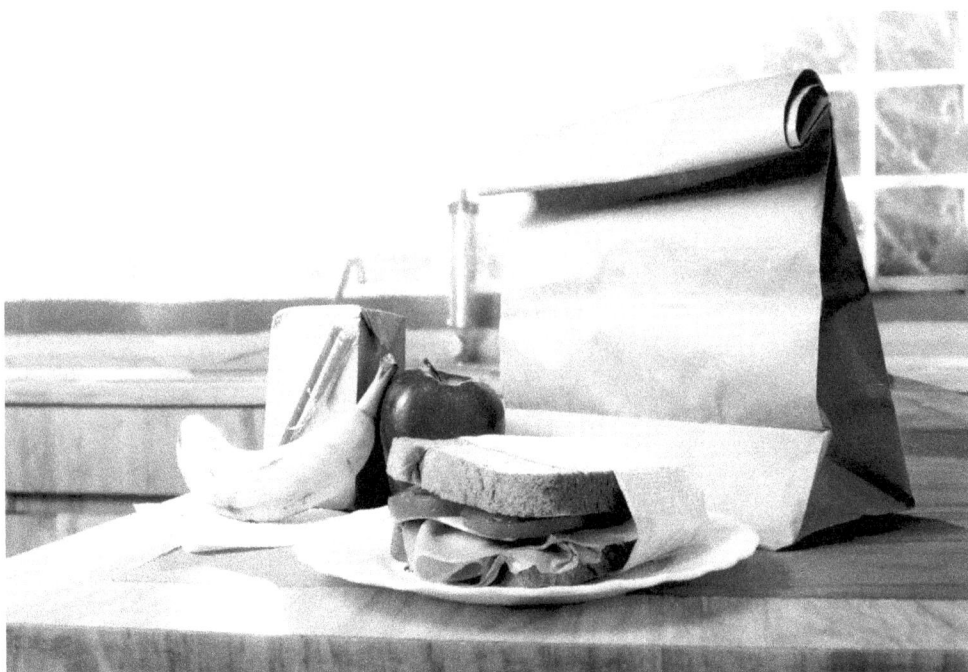

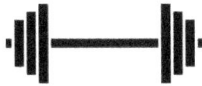

P art of counting macros and the Junk Food Fit program is meal prep, but meal prep isn't about plastic Tupperware containers and the same monotonous meals all week. Meal prep isn't even about eating dry chicken breast and flavorless rice.

Meal prep is about taking control of your life. It's about taking time out of your busy schedule to actually pack your meal ahead of time instead of buying fast food every day or grabbing a packaged microwaveable meal on your way out the door.

Moreover, meal prep is about going back to the simpler times when mom stayed at home in her sundress cooking and cleaning and dad went to work in his coveralls to the coal mines. When kids actually ran outside to play. When we had enough time to care about ourselves and make our own dinner. A simpler time when we didn't have to rely on McDonalds and Chipotle to keep our tanks full as we run through our overly hectic, nonstop, workaholic days.

meal prep is easy

What is meal prep? Meal prep is just a fancy term for "packing your lunch." It's nothing to be afraid of.

Whether you call it meal prep or packing your lunch, the organized behavior is all about *you*. It's about making meals that fit *your* lifestyle and satisfy *your* palette. If you're preparing for a bodybuilding competition then maybe yes, you need to eat very structured meals of chicken and rice for long periods of time. But most people are just looking for a way to lose a little weight, keep it off, and love how they look. Love how they feel. To do this, you can still eat what you love, but you might have to eat a little bit less of it, or at the least, not eat it every day.

If you've never meal prepped before, the **first** thing I suggest you do is buy containers in which you can take your food to work (or school or wherever). This can be Tupperware, plastic sandwich bags, aluminum foil—all depending on your preference and meal plan. There is no need for special containers, just go to Target or the local grocery store and buy a cheap pack of six to start. Once you get going, you might find that you prefer a specific color or style, so start small in case you change your preferences later.

Secondly, you need to figure out how much food you should pack each day (your calories and your macros). The USDA has calculated approximate values of calorie intake as shown in the chart on the next page, varying by gender and age, and ranging from 1600 calories for elderly females to 3200 calories for active, young adult males.

While the chart is a great place to start and a great guideline, it's not perfect. Calorie expenditure varies depending on gender, age, height, weight, muscle mass, physical activity, genetics, and it's key to learn *your* personal calorie needs—which can also change throughout your lifetime based on your daily habits.

This and other great information, including the newest Dietary Guidelines and Food Fact Sheets, can be found on the USDA Center for Nutrition Policy and Promotion's website (http://www.cnpp.usda.gov).

Estimated Calorie Needs per Day by Age, Gender, and Physical Activity Level

Activity level	Male			Female		
	Sedentary	Moderately active	Active	Sedentary	Moderately active	Active
Age (years)						
2	1000	1000	1000	1000	1000	1000
3	1200	1400	1400	1000	1200	1400
4	1200	1400	1600	1200	1400	1400
5	1200	1400	1600	1200	1400	1600
6	1400	1600	1800	1200	1400	1600
7	1400	1600	1800	1200	1600	1800
8	1400	1600	2000	1400	1600	1800
9	1600	1800	2000	1400	1600	1800
10	1600	1800	2200	1400	1800	2000
11	1800	2000	2200	1600	1800	2000
12	1800	2200	2400	1600	2000	2200
13	2000	2200	2600	1600	2000	2200
14	2000	2400	2800	1800	2000	2400
15	2200	2600	3000	1800	2000	2400
16	2400	2800	3200	1800	2000	2400
17	2400	2800	3200	1800	2000	2400
18	2400	2800	3200	1800	2000	2400
19-20	2600	2800	3000	2000	2200	2400
21-25	2400	2800	3000	2000	2200	2400
26-30	2400	2600	3000	1800	2000	2400
31-35	2400	2600	3000	1800	2000	2200
36-40	2400	2600	2800	1800	2000	2200
41-45	2200	2600	2800	1800	2000	2200
46-50	2200	2400	2800	1800	2000	2200
51-55	2200	2400	2800	1600	1800	2200
56-60	2200	2400	2600	1600	1800	2200
61-65	2000	2400	2600	1600	1800	2000
66-70	2000	2200	2600	1600	1800	2000
71-75	2000	2200	2600	1600	1800	2000
76+	2000	2200	2400	1600	1800	2000

Aside from using this chart, my suggestion would be to download a calorie-counting app for your phone (*e.g.* MyFitnessPal), input your body stats, and find out how many calories you **need** each day. This should be the amount of calories your body needs in order to maintain your current weight (based on your height, weight, age, exercise level, etc.). Compare the value from the app to the value in the chart—they should be similar.

You can also use a calorie-counting website, but then it's harder to keep track of your calories throughout the day if any snacks or meals should change.

After you know how many calories your body **needs,** then you can choose a calorie level less than that for weight loss. Some calorie-counters calculate this for you.

These counters are usually pretty accurate, but you should test the number out for yourself by weighing yourself each day. If you consume the **need** number and your weight does not fluctuate much, then you are probably right on the money. If the weight continues to move up (or down) one day to another for multiple days in a row, you may need to make adjustments.

Remember that no two people are the same, and what works for your neighbor may not work for you, so adjust as necessary; your journey is your journey, so play around with your numbers and find out what works for you.

However, any medical issues may interfere with the accurateness of the calculator. It's best to consult your doctor but to also weigh yourself frequently in the beginning to be sure.

Slow and steady wins the race!

When reducing calories, start slowly! The last thing you want is to starve yourself; if your calorie intake level is set too low, you might get discouraged and think, "I can't do this."

Instead, you should calculate the amount of calories you ate *yesterday* and *the day before* (don't cheat!). Use those numbers to determine the average calorie intake that you are currently consuming, prior to any thoughts of reducing your food intake.

Ok, now if that number is higher than your **need** number from the previous page, reduce it by 100 calories. Shoot for 100 less than what you normally consume, and see how that feels. Once you are ok with that, reduce it again and again until you eventually reach your **need** value. The last thing you want to do is go from 3000 down to 1600 calories cold turkey: this will discourage you and will make the process much more difficult.

Alternatively, if the number you typically consume in a day is lower than your **need** number, increase your intake to meet your body's needs. Sometimes eating too few calories can impede weight loss because the body is then struggling to find fuel. *Remember to always consult your doctor when changing your diet and altering your caloric intake.*

In terms of macros, an adult who isn't concerned with eating a lot of protein should stick to about a 60% carb diet, 30% fat, and 10% protein.[18] The recent Dietary Guidelines recommends macro ranges rather than finite targets, as shown in the table to the right.

Once you start working out and decide to increase your protein intake, the typical recommendation in the weight lifting world is *one gram* of protein for every pound that you weigh. For me, my diet would then consist of 33% protein,

Dietary Guidelines for Americans 2015-2020		
	% min	% max
Carbs	45%	65%
Protein	10%	35%
Fat	20%	35%

then I would split the rest with carbs and fat. This weight lifting method could have you consuming 100+ grams of protein per day, while the FDA recommends a daily value of only 50 grams protein for an adult. The extra amount ensures you have enough proteins in your body to function properly and then to have extra that can be used to build muscle.

Aside from protein, the FDA recommends a daily value of 300 grams carbohydrates and 65 grams of fat (this translates to the 60% carbs and 30% fat as previously stated).[18] You will find some weight loss methods that suggest to keep your fat percent much lower, while others suggest keeping your carbs lower.[19] You should try out different percentages on your own because different macro levels work better or worse depending on the person (your age, weight, metabolism, activity, etc).

Remember that you always want to have a diet with all three macros: carbs, protein, and fat. They all play important roles in a proper functioning body.

Listen to your body!

When you start on this Junk Food Fit journey, pay close attention to your body and your food cravings as you change your caloric intake. Over time, your fullness state will change once you give your body enough practice at that new calorie amount. Eventually you will eat two slices instead of four slices of pizza and be amazed at how full you feel. In order to notice a difference, though, you have to pay attention. Take control of your eating and focus on the goals you set for yourself.

Now that you know how many calories to eat each day, the **third** thing you need to do for meal prep is PREP. Prepare your meals ahead of time. This can mean you cook all your meals for the week on Sunday, pack them, and store them away in the freezer, or this can mean you cook every night for the following day. Depending on your own schedule and how fresh you want your meals to be, you choose your favorite option.

Yet, if you truly are too bogged down to make all your own food yourself, there are plenty of meal prep service companies available now (*e.g.* FitFuelPrep, FuelMeals). Take advantage of their healthy and convenient meals when you need to!

Lastly, eat! There's no point in preparing your meals if you aren't going to eat them. Make food that you love and that doesn't make your skin crawl. Take your Tupperware containers with you to work (or wherever you are going); it might be helpful to buy a cooler to put them in, since you might be taking three or more containers with you (*e.g.* 6 Pack bag, FitMark bag).

Just because meal prep is usually associated with packing single serve containers for your own lunches for the week, it doesn't have to end there. Meal prep doesn't have to be solely about preparing your lunches to take to work. Meal prep can also mean cooking dinner for your family. Baking cookies on the weekend. It might take two hours to make a good meal, but if you have two hours to binge watch episodes of your favorite TV series, then you have two hours to cook instead of eat out.

If you don't already have a television in your kitchen, put one in there! You can do two things at once. My mother always used to cook us dinner and watch the news at the same time. With a TV set in the kitchen, now the only thing you would be compromising is the comfort of your couch—but that will always be there for you when you're done!

Remember—let's Bring Back the Cookie Jar! #CookieJar

Want to Count CALORIES?

Let's go through an example.

Susie wants to lose weight. She is 28 years old and works a desk job, then comes home and watches television the rest of the night with her roommate.

Weight: **180 lbs**
Age: **28**
Average daily calories: **2250+**

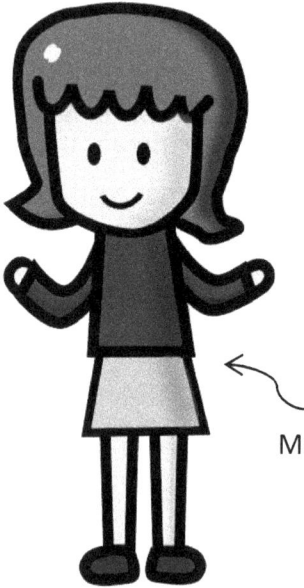

Nearly every day, Susie drinks coffee, eats an egg and cheese bagel for breakfast, a turkey sandwich and yogurt for lunch, snacks at her desk all day, then comes home and eats take-out for dinner, mostly pizza or chinese food with a soda or beer.

By using the chart, we find that a 28 year-old like Susie should be eating **1800** calories each day.

She started off the day with 400 calories in her bagel. Her lunch only costs her 350 calories, but the take-out and beer is at least 1000 calories. The candy bar she snacked on and the pack of Twizzlers

Meet Susie!

Breakfast: 400 cals

Lunch: 350 cals

Dinner: 1000 cals

+ Snacks: 500 cals

Total: 2250+ cals

added up to another 500 calories, not to mention the sugar and milk she used in her coffee in the morning. Very easily, Susie's simple day added up to 2250+ calories!

Since she is clearly over her limit, her first step was to knock down 100 calories from her diet. She stopped eating Twizzlers, reaching about 2100 calories. She stayed at this level for a few days, then felt ready to move down again.

She then made an easy change and drank water with her dinner instead of the soda or beer. This brought down her number again to about 2000 calories.

After finally feeling ready to make the full adjustment, Susie starting making her own dinner and aimed for a total 1800 calories. The gradual takedown of her calories helped her stay on track and never discouraged her.

She also weighed herself a few times per week and realized that at the 1800 level, she remained at a consistent 170/171 lbs.

Susie's experience is just one example of how things could be

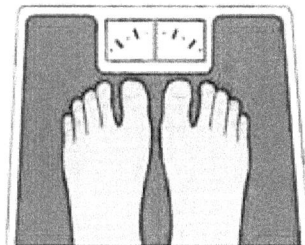

Susie's Weight

Day 1: 180 lbs

Day 6: 179 lbs

Day 13: 178 lbs

Day 19: 177 lbs

Day 25: 177 lbs

Day 30: 175 lbs

Day 44: 173 lbs

Day 56: 170 lbs

Day 59: 171 lbs

Day 62: 170 lbs

done. If she wanted to keep eating what she was eating (pizza, beer, etc.), she could have started exercising—changing her sedentary lifestyle to a moderately active lifestyle. This new activity would automatically increase her 1800 recommended calorie amount to 2000-2400, depending. She could have also changed her eating habits altogether, but by taking things out one by one, she allowed her body to adjust without acting too drastically.

Want to Count MACROS?

Let's go through an example.

Johnny wants to lose weight. He is 45 years old and is a stay-at-home daddy.

Weight: **250 lbs**

Age: **45**

Average daily calories: **1500**

Meet Johnny!

Johnny considers himself moderately active since he is busy with the kids all day. By using the chart he finds that he often does not eat enough food!

While Johnny eats plenty on the weekends, some weekdays he might only eat 1500 calories, staying too busy and sometimes forgetting to eat! His new calorie amount is **2600**.

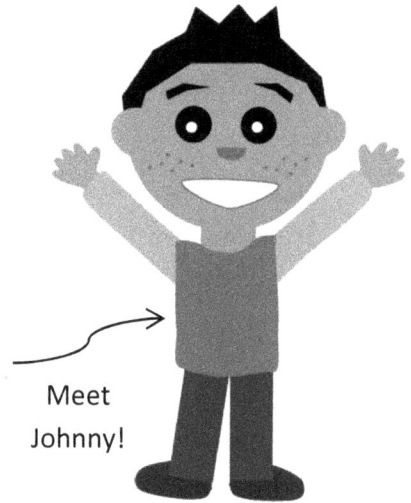

Breakfast: 250 cals

Lunch: what lunch?

Dinner: 1000 cals

+ Snacks: 250 cals

Total: 1500 cals

Johnny wants to use the macro method so he can eat whatever his kids have to eat. He also decided to start working out everyday while the kids take a nap.

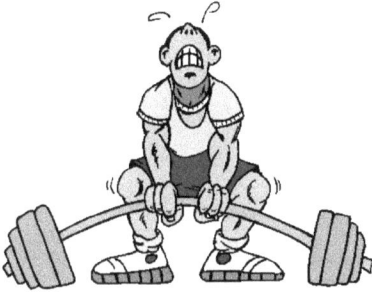

Johnny's macros

38% of 2600 calories

= 1000 cals from protein

= 250 grams protein

31% of 2600 calories

= 800 cals from carbs

= 200 grams carbs

31% of 2600 calories

= 800 cals from fat

= 89 grams fat

He wants to eat 1 gram of protein per pound he weighs, so that would equal 250 grams of protein. Since there are 4 calories per gram of protein, that equals 1000 calories from protein—or about 38% of his total calories. Hence, his macro breakdown is 38/31/31 protein, carb, fat.

Now whenever he eats something, he enters it into his food tracker on his phone. He always aims to reach 250 total grams of protein, 200 grams carbs, and about 89 grams of fat each day.

After time, he noticed that his weight reduced even though he increased his intake from 1500 calories to 2600! He never realized how much it matters to eat... and he never skipped lunch agan!

More on Macros...

The key to macro dieting and Junk Food Fit is not only evaluating the *calorie content* of a food, but also the *MACRO* breakdown of a food.

For example, one large apple contains about:
110 calories, 29 g Carbs, 0 g protein, 0 g fat

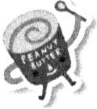

Two tablespoons peanut butter contains about:
190 calories, 6 g carb, 7 g protein, 16 g fat

One donut contains about:
240 calories, 29 g Carbs, 2 g protein, 15 g fat

If you ate a breakfast consisting of an apple and two tablespoons of peanut butter, your total for that meal would be:

Apple + peanut butter =
300 calories, 35 g Carb, 7 g protein, 16 g fat

So in theory, you could eat a donut instead of the apple and peanut butter, and still be okay. While the calories are not exactly the same, the **donut** brings in fewer carbs (29 vs. 35), similar fat (15 vs. 16), but not as much protein (2 vs. 7).

In a diet high in protein, this is a downside because you always want to opt for the option with the most protein. But, because we all know that it's hard to stay away from the yummy goodness that are donuts, cakes, candy, chocolate, yummy yummy yummy Mmmmmmmmmm .... ☺ there has to be a way to keep them in your diet, as long as everything else in your diet is on point (you can always add an extra ounce of chicken to your dinner later that day to make up for the protein).

This is not an excuse for you to eat donuts every day though! While macro dieting is supposed to allow you to fit in "bad" food in your diet, you should still be conscious of the fact that the apple and the peanut butter is overall the healthier choice (vitamins, minerals, fiber, etc.).

In addition, there are pros and cons to monitoring your food intake this way. Of course, the benefit is that you can still have your favorite snacks here and there as long as you don't over-indulge. The bad part about this is that *if you can't control yourself* one donut might turn into a whole box of donuts!

Tip: Keep track of your food as the day goes along. That way if you have a slice of cake at your coworker's retirement party, you can remove the cup of rice that you were supposed to eat for lunch and swap it out for a cup of spinach instead (and still stay on track).

Now you try!

Check your calories!
See how you are doing with your food!
Get some help with meal choices!

Step One: Where are you now?

Gender: _____ Age: ____ Weight: _____ Height: _____

What did you eat yesterday (or today)?

Column A	Column B		Column C		Column D
Food	**# servings**		**Calories per serving**		**Total Calories (Columns B*C)**
ex. pizza	2 slices	x	350 per slice	=	700
		x		=	
		x		=	
		x		=	
		x		=	
		x		=	
		x		=	
		x		=	
		x		=	
		x		=	
		x		=	
		x		=	
		x		=	

Determine your **current** number. Add it all up (Column D),
how many calories did you eat throughout the entire day? _____
*there are more of these worksheets in the back of the book to use if needed

Step Two: Where should you be?

Gender: _____ Age: ____ Weight: _____ Height: _____

Use the chart below to determine how many calories you **should** be eating each day:

Estimated Calorie Needs per Day by Age, Gender, and Physical Activity Level

Activity level	Male			Female		
	Sedentary	Moderately active	Active	Sedentary	Moderately active	Active
Age (years)						
15	2200	2600	3000	1800	2000	2400
16	2400	2800	3200	1800	2000	2400
17	2400	2800	3200	1800	2000	2400
18	2400	2800	3200	1800	2000	2400
19-20	2600	2800	3000	2000	2200	2400
21-25	2400	2800	3000	2000	2200	2400
26-30	2400	2600	3000	1800	2000	2400
31-35	2400	2600	3000	1800	2000	2200
36-40	2400	2600	2800	1800	2000	2200
41-45	2200	2600	2800	1800	2000	2200
46-50	2200	2400	2800	1800	2000	2200
51-55	2200	2400	2800	1600	1800	2200
56-60	2200	2400	2600	1600	1800	2200
61-65	2000	2400	2600	1600	1800	2000
66-70	2000	2200	2600	1600	1800	2000
71-75	2000	2200	2600	1600	1800	2000
76+	2000	2200	2400	1600	1800	2000

Record the amount you **should** be eating here: _____

Compare that number to your current number from Step One.

Are you eating more calories than you should be? Are you eating less?
*Remember that this **should** number could be off slightly, but it is a good place to start.

Step Three: How do I get to where I want to be?

Record your **current** calorie intake here: _____   *example: 4000*

Record your **should** value here: _____   *example: 2200*

If you aren't eating enough, simply increase your intake to the **should** value. If you are eating too much, start off by reducing your **current** calorie intake by a small amount, working your way toward the **should** amount. In the example (4000 and 2200 calories), we will drop the calorie intake down to 3500. If your difference isn't as drastic as this case, maybe only reduce by 50 or 100 calories to start.

Example new intake amount: 3500 calories
For a few weeks, keep track of the foods you eat. Cut small things here and there (replace soda with water, mayonnaise with low-fat mayonnaise). Keep track of your weight and how you feel.

Once you are confident at 3500 calories and are ready to move on, reduce again. In this case, we will reduce to 3000 calories. Depending on your own case, you may want to reduce by only 50 or 100 calories.

Example new intake amount: 3000 calories
Keep track of all your foods and how you feel. Eventually you will see the difference in your body and your attitude, and you will want to reduce your calories once again.

After a few more weeks and reductions in your calories, you will eventually be at the **should** value. For this instance, we finally reached 2200 calories.

Example new intake amount: 2200 calories
You are now at your **should** value. Stay at the amount for a while and keep track of your weight. You may be okay staying at that amount, but depending on your progress, you can go below that amount to keep losing weight as well. Just be careful not to go too far below because then you won't be consuming enough, and your body will go into "starvation mode." We don't want that!

All in all...
You have to be ready mentally when losing weight. To go cold turkey and jump quickly from 4000 to 2200 calories will not only be a shock to your system and body, but a shock to your routine. It's best to reduce slowly; otherwise, you will be hungry and want to give up. Small changes make all the difference—after all, it has to be a **lifestyle** change, not a temporary change!

Sample meal plan

Don't know where to start?

Here's a sample meal plan (*if you haven't already, make sure you buy a food scale to weigh out your food so you know exactly how much you are eating!)

Meal	Food	Calories
Breakfast	½ cup oatmeal	150
	Protein shake (1 scoop protein powder+water)	120
Snack	1 medium sized apple	80
	2 Tablespoons peanut butter	190
Lunch (**tuna salad wrap**)	Two cans tuna	200
	1 whole wheat wrap	110
	1 container Greek yogurt, non-fat, unsweetened	90
	Lettuce or spinach	5
Snack (salad)	2 cups mixed greens	15
	1 tablespoon shredded cheese	55
	1 tablespoon salad dressing	45
	2 ounces grilled chicken	55
Dinner	6 oz. ground turkey	230
	1 cup steamed broccoli	30
	1 cup white rice	242
	2 teaspoons olive oil sprinkled on top	120
Snack	Protein bar	190
	Total calories =	1927

*adjust as necessary to meet desired total calories

Sample meal plan

Meal	Food	Calories
Breakfast	Egg white omelet using 6 egg whites	102
	1 banana	110
	1 Tablespoon peanut butter	95
Snack	1 clementine	35
	1 serving almonds	160
Lunch (turkey eggplant lasagna)	Ground turkey	200
	Eggplant	60
	Tomato sauce	60
	Greek yogurt, non-fat, unsweetened	90
	Fat free cheese	25
Snack	Protein shake (1 scoop protein powder+milk)	210
Dinner	6 oz. salmon	354
	1 cup steamed kale	30
	3 oz. sweet potatoes	110
Snack	Protein bar	190
	2 tablespoons non-fat whipping crème	25
	Total calories =	1856

*adjust as necessary to meet desired total calories

Sample meal plan

Meal	Food	Calories
Breakfast	Protein bar	190
	2 slices whole wheat bread	140
	1 Tablespoon peanut butter	95
Snack	1 container Greek yogurt, non-fat, unsweetened	90
	1 cup blueberries	83
Lunch	8 oz. lean ground turkey	306
	Fat free cheese	25
	1 cup white rice	242
	1 cup steamed green beans	44
Snack	Protein shake (1 scoop protein powder+water)	120
Dinner	14 extra-large cooked shrimp	160
	1 cup sliced cucumber	16
	1 cup pasta	200
Snack	1 Tablespoon peanut butter	95
	4 tablespoons Non-fat whipped crème	50

Total calories =   1806

*adjust as necessary to meet desired total calories

Shrimp and Spaghetti Squash

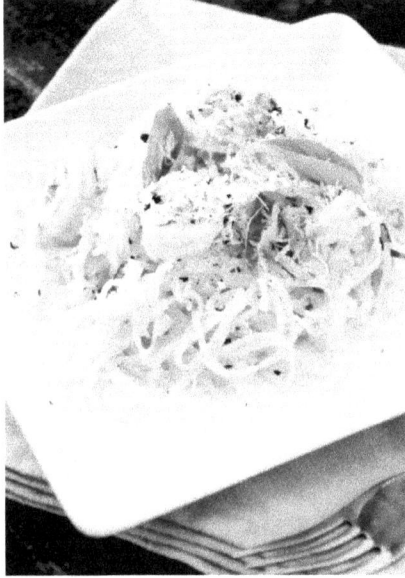

1. Cut the squash open into halves or quarters.
2. Heat in the microwave or in the oven.
3. Once cooked, scrape with a fork to pull the squash apart.
4. Open a bag of pre-cooked shrimp.
5. Sautee the shrimp with ½ tablespoon olive oil.

Single serve – about 11 medium sized shrimp and one cup squash (add ½ cup spinach if you want some greens).

Fish and Asparagus

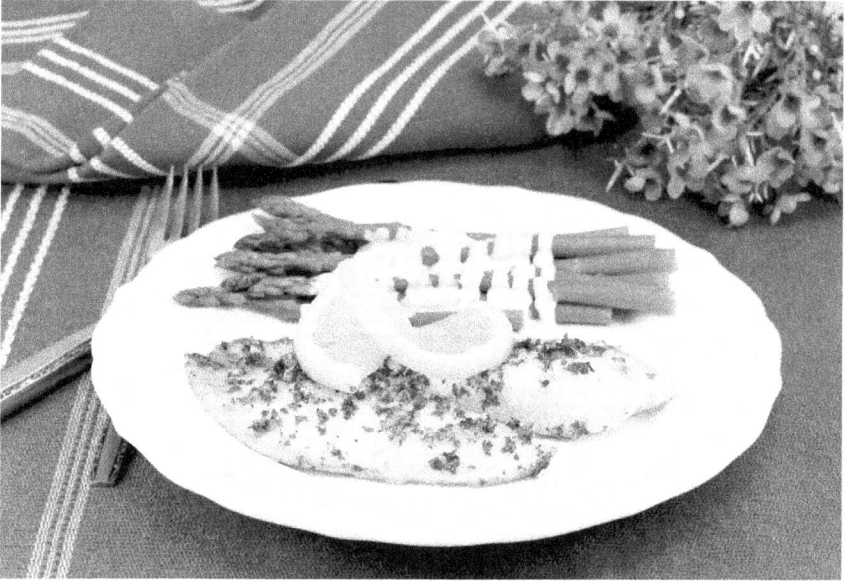

1. Sautee the fish (cod or tilapia) with ½ tablespoon olive oil.
2. In separate pan, cook the asparagus spears with water or ½ tablespoon olive oil.
3. Squeeze lemon slice over your dish for flavor.
4. If desired, use mustard or a low-calorie sauce on the side.

Single serve – about one large fillet of fish (or two medium fillets) and 10 spears of asparagus.

Tuna Salad Wrap

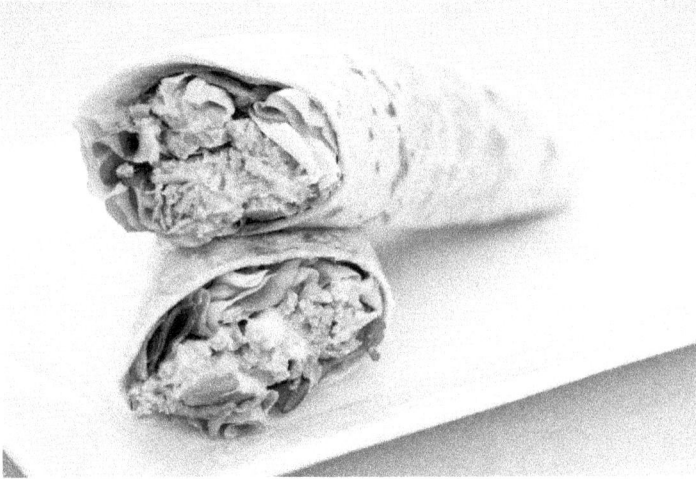

1. Open two cans of tuna.
2. Mix with ¼ cup nonfat (or low-fat), plain Greek yogurt. Add another ¼ cup yogurt if too dry.
3. Season with cilantro, salt, and pepper.
4. Scoop into a wrap, add some lettuce, and eat!

Serving – makes one or two wraps, depending on how filled you like your wraps!

Turkey Zucchini Lasagna

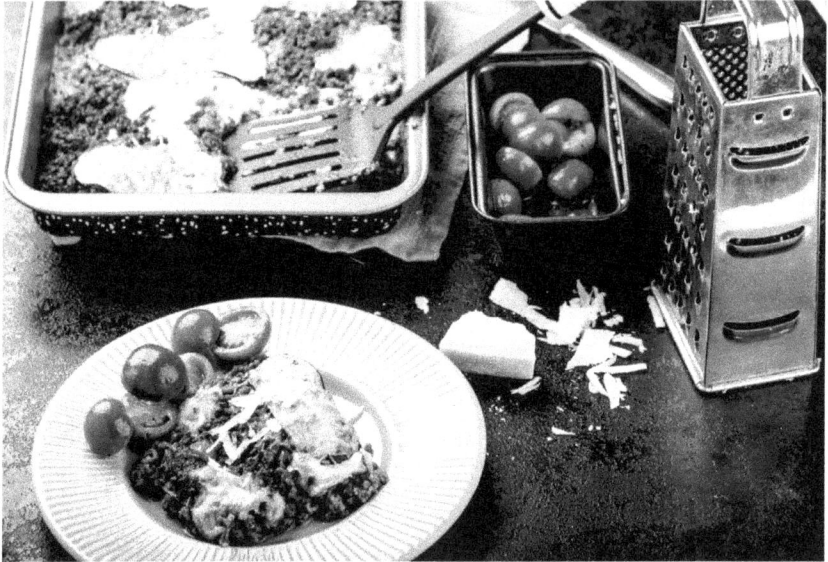

1. On stove, add ½ cup water to pan and one pack (about 16 ounces) 93% ground turkey. Cook until well-done.
2. Cut zucchini (or eggplant) in to thin strips.
3. In lasagna pan, prepare similarly to regular lasagna using red pasta sauce, zucchini or eggplant (instead of pasta), and cooked ground turkey.
4. Use Greek yogurt instead of ricotta cheese on each layer.
5. On the top layer, sprinkle with low-fat cheddar cheese.
6. Cover pan with aluminum foil.
7. Bake in oven at 425°F for 30 minutes. Remove cover and bake for an additional 10 minutes.

Single serve – one or two squares lasagna.

Chicken, Rice, and Broccoli

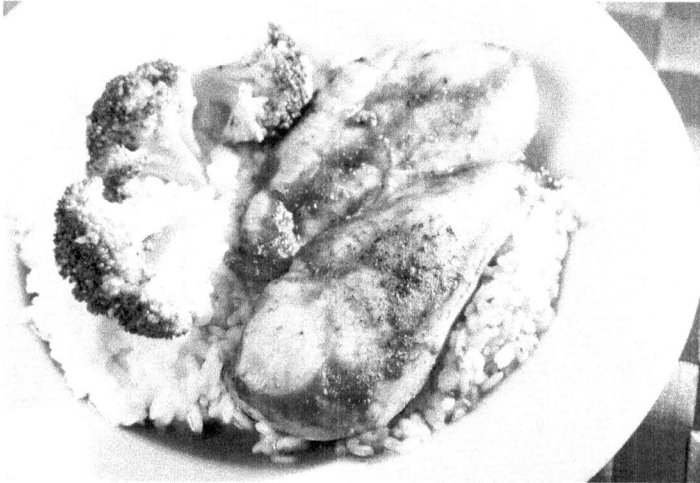

1. Broil chicken breasts in the oven at 425°F for 90 minutes or until well-done.
2. Make white rice (or brown) in pot on the stove.
3. Steam the broccoli in pot on the stove.
4. Add some olive oil (one teaspoon) for flavor.
5. Add seasonings as you desire.

Single serve – one chicken breast, one cup rice, and one cup greens.

Egg Whites with Avocado Toast

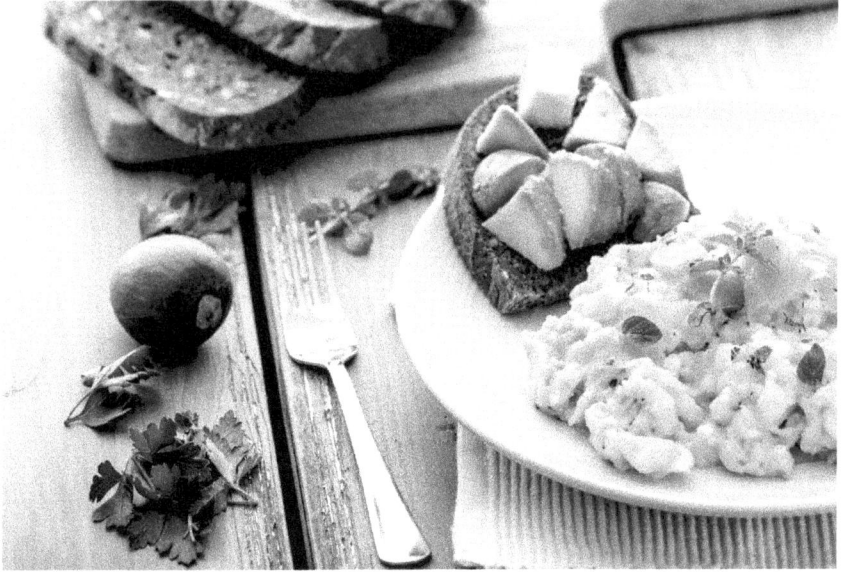

1. Grease a skillet with cooking spray.
2. Separate 6 egg whites from the shell and cook on the stove on low heat.
3. *For added color and flavor, use one whole egg in addition to the whites.*
4. Cut avocado in half and remove the pit. Slice the avocado.
5. Toast pieces of whole wheat bread in the toaster.

Single serve – 6 egg whites (or 4 whites and one whole egg), ¼ avocado, and two slices of toast.

CHAPTER ELEVEN

Key Foods

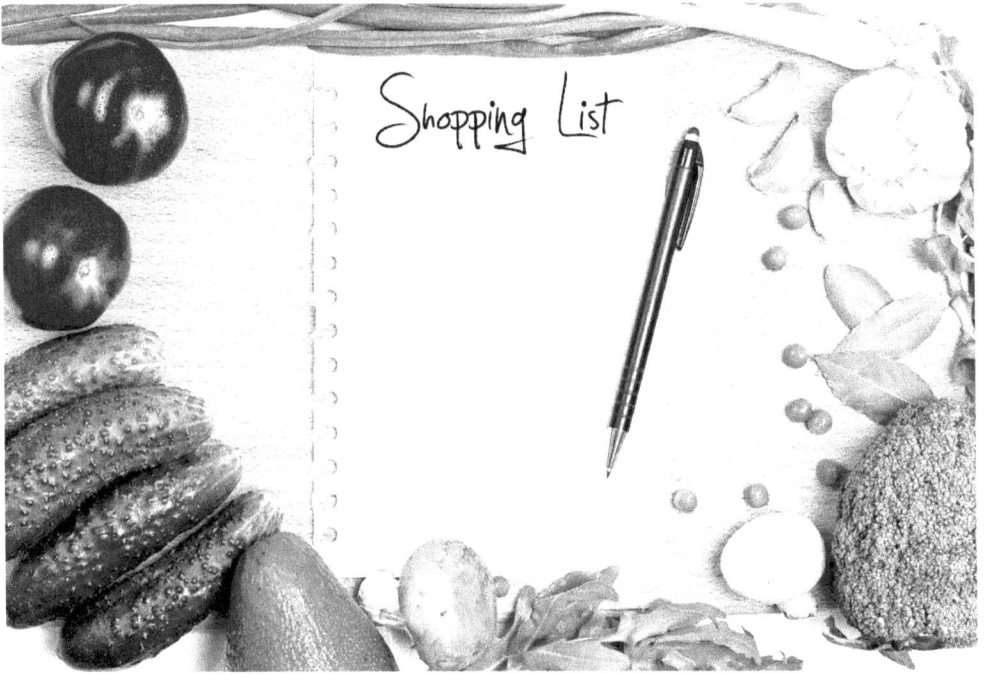

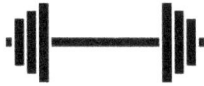

It's important that we make the transition from *old you* to *new you* as simple and as painless as possible. By taking control of the foods you ingest and by making use of your own kitchen, natural weight loss will take place.

Logically, if you replace fatty, fast food with freshly grilled and cooked foods, the caloric intake should be less. On top of that, when you prepare your own food, you will start to understand exactly *what* you are putting in your body.

Also, by keeping track of your calories, you will begin to notice how many excess sugars are in prepared foods that you might buy at the grocery store; you can make the same product in your home without extra sugars, salts, and processing aids.

Now that you know a little bit about the pre-made food purchased at grocery stores and restaurants and you are equipped with necessary tools to choose better foods, I want to provide you with a list of some foods that should always be in your pantry. This convenient list should help jumpstart you into healthier eating habits and patterns of more home cooking.

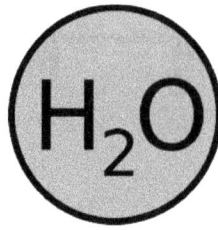

H₂O

wATER!!!!

Water is the first thing on the list, and it gets its own page because it is just *that* important. Either invest in a water bottle that you can carry around with you at all times and refill, or buy bottled water so you can grab one quickly on your way out the door.

Always have some type of water source near you. Even at night, keep a bottle on your nightstand in case you wake up at midnight with a dry mouth. Ward off the parched feeling by drinking a sip when you wake up first thing in the morning too.

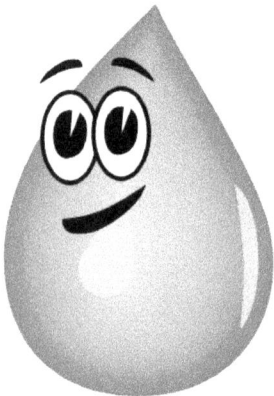

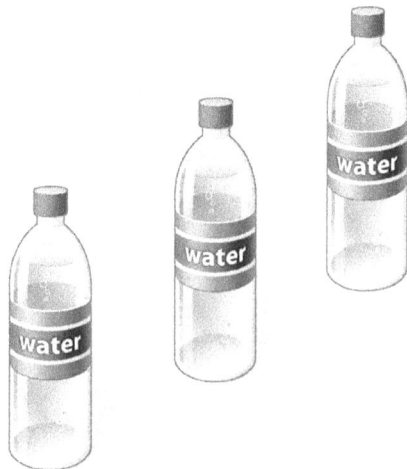

Shopping List

The rest of the list is minutely important compared to water. The food options you have are endless, but some key foods that are great to have in your kitchen at all times are listed below. These are go-to items that can be used to make a meal without much forethought.

✓ Whole wheat bread
✓ Whole wheat wraps
✓ Rice—brown or white
✓ Oatmeal
✓ Potatoes and sweet potatoes
✓ Eggs (in shell)
✓ Egg whites (liquid)
✓ Deli meats (chicken, turkey)
✓ Meats—chicken, turkey, fish (ground, breast, steak)
✓ Fresh fruits
✓ Greens—fresh, frozen, or canned
✓ Peanut butter
✓ Condiments—ketchup, mustard, fat-free salad dressings
✓ Fat-free sour cream
✓ Fat-free whipped cream
✓ Seasonings (like Mrs. Dash)
✓ Protein powder

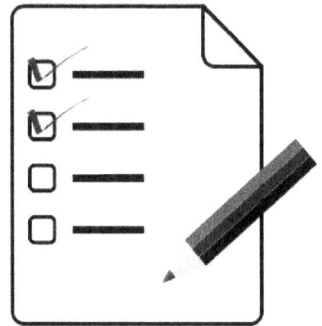

Baking List

In addition, if you are baking or cooking meals from scratch, it's important to have, at minimum, these ingredients readily available:

- ✓ Whole wheat flour
- ✓ All-purpose flour
- ✓ Brown sugar
- ✓ White sugar
- ✓ Eggs (in shell)
- ✓ Cocoa powder
- ✓ Baking soda
- ✓ Baking powder
- ✓ Coconut oil, olive oil, vegetable oil
- ✓ Cooking spray
- ✓ Salt
- ✓ Cinnamon
- ✓ Vanilla extract

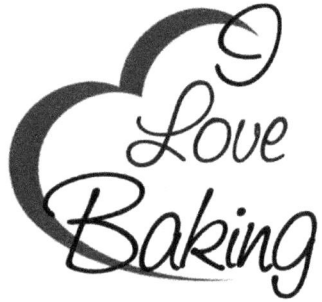

Besides these ingredients, you should also get your hands on a hand mixer, measuring spoons, measuring cups (both liquid and powder), mixing bowls, mixing spoons, rolling pin, wax paper, and a few spatulas of varying sizes.

With what you have read so far, you are now equipped with (a) the basic knowledge to prepare you for a trip to the grocery store as well as the (b) baking/cooking tools for your tool belt to enable you to create some great meals for you and your family. The only thing that's left is the ***exercise!***

CHAPTER TWELVE

Keep Moving!

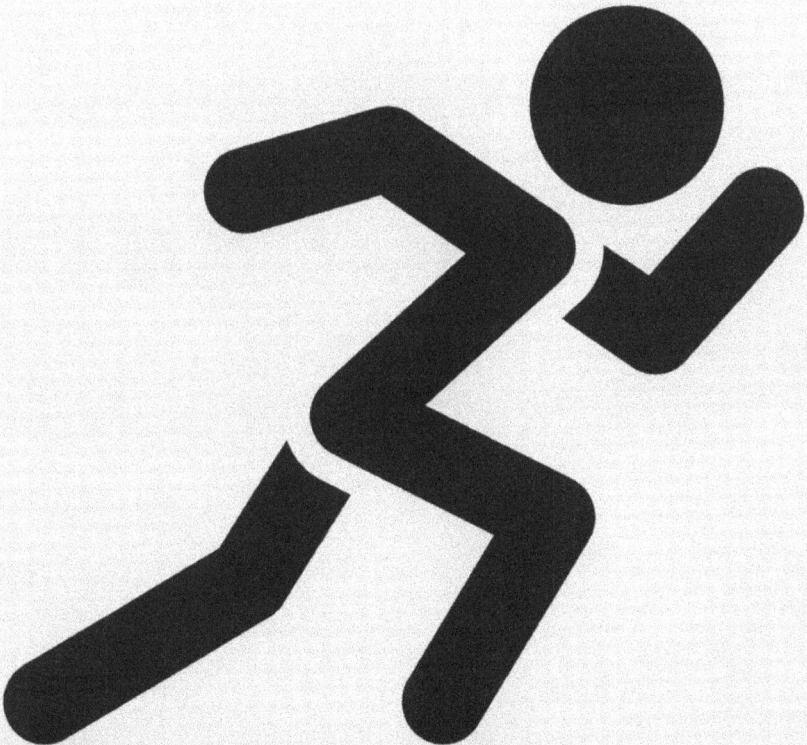

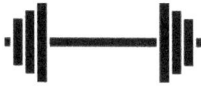

When it comes to working out, you should look at it this way: if there were a zombie apocalypse tomorrow, **could you outrun them?**

As a food science and nutrition professor, I've heard all sorts of questions ranging from, "Should I throw away an egg if it has a blood spot on it?" to "Does juicing kill vitamins in the fruits and vegetables?" The best questions are the ones from people outside the classroom who are interested in learning more about food and what I do for a living.

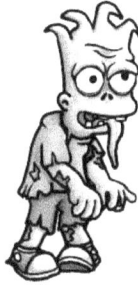

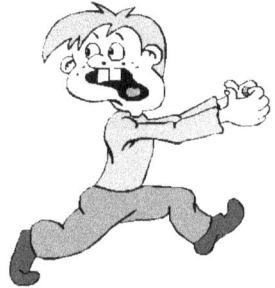

One day I was leaving my classroom after teaching, and one of the janitors at the university started talking to me. She asked if I taught nutrition, and if I could help her lose weight. I told her a few things, telling her that it's a combination of watching what you eat and also doing some exercise, even if just a little bit. I also mentioned that she should simply start walking a short distance each day for exercise, nothing big, just start small. The rest of the conversation went something like this:

She said, "Oh, my knees hurt when I walk and run. So I can't exercise."

I responded, "I understand. So instead of walking, work out in the pool. There's less impact on your joints."

"I don't know how to swim."

"Ok. Let's focus on your food then if you don't have many exercise options."

She nodded her head, "Ok what do you suggest?"

"Well, take out some of the sweets. Candies, cookies, cakes. Stuff like that."

She made a face and said, "I don't know. But I like cake too much."

At the end of it all, I chuckled and didn't know what else to say. So I wished her a good night and kept walking to my car.

Excuses are easy to make. If you're not willing to put the effort into your *lifestyle* change, your *body* won't change. If you don't attack the weed from the root, it's going to keep growing, no matter how many times you cut the stem.

But you're in luck! Change is easy when you start small. Start slowly! Even a simple walk each day is better than nothing. A small change is better than no change at all, and that small change could be the beginning of a tremendous transformation.

Six-pack abs takes time and effort!

When it comes to making a lifestyle change, you must be in it for the long game. You must realize that weight loss will not happen overnight; this lifestyle change should be permanent.

Especially in the U.S., it can be tough to make a lifestyle change because we have grown so accustomed to eating out and always having soda and candy in our pantries. Outings with friends revolve around brunch and mimosas or kegs and eggs. Even holidays celebrate the abundance of food that we as

Americans should be thankful for. In making this lifestyle change, **you have to want it.**

It's all about *you.* You have to be ready to make the change. You have to be ready to go on this journey alone. Similar to how you can choose your car, choose your clothes, choose your boyfriend or girlfriend; you can choose your food. But you have to be strong and be prepared for people to question your methods.

Why don't you want cake? It's Amy's birthday.

Why do you bring so much food with you to work?

How come you choose to go to the gym instead of joining us for dinner?

You don't hang out with us anymore. Do you not like us?

With the lifestyle change, your **priorities** will change over time. If you truly want to lose weight and maintain a great shape, you need to understand that the lifestyle change encompasses both food and exercise. While abs may be made in the kitchen, you won't stay away from the keg belly if you don't start moving too!

By using the tools you've learned about food in this book, you are one step closer to making that lifestyle change and becoming a newer fitter you. Along with the food, though, make sure to **keep moving!** Train with your trainer, workout by yourself too. Move whenever you can. Choose the stairs over the elevator. Park away from the door so you can walk across the parking lot. Play outside with your kids. Whatever opportunity presents itself to move, **do it!**

Keep moving, and while doing so, remember to follow the same motto as our food plans: variety with consistency. In the beginning, it doesn't really matter whether you choose weight lifting, the treadmill, elliptical, or even group classes as your exercise, it's just important that you start. As you grow and become less of a beginner, you can learn to optimize your workouts. And last but not least, remember to reward yourself with a homemade cookie every once in a while (as long as it fits in your macros) because you Brought Back the Cookie Jar! #CookieJar

CHAPTER THIRTEEN

Recipes

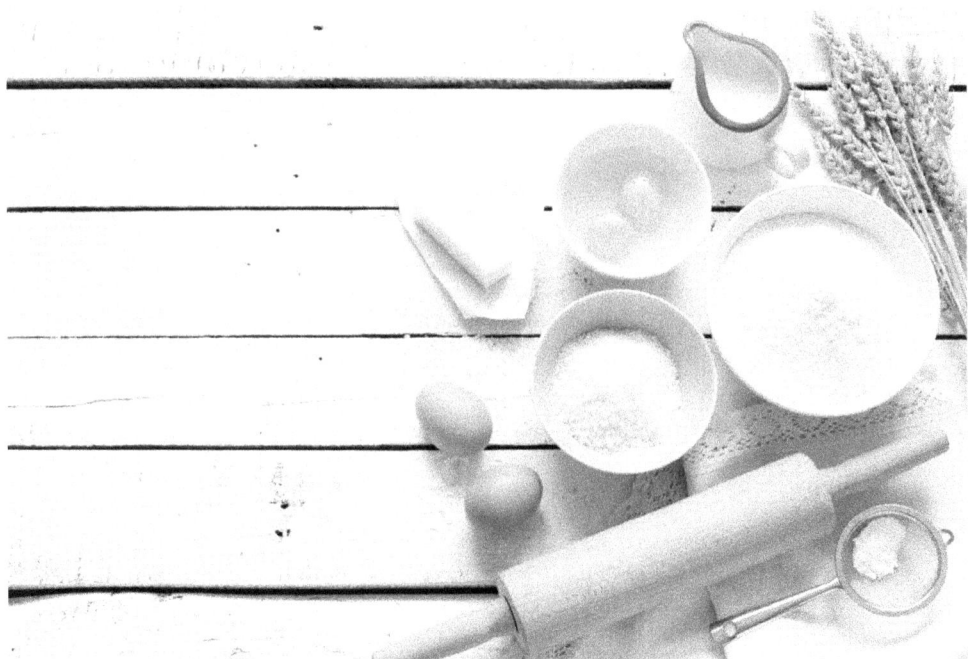

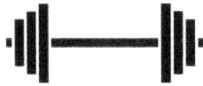

L et's bring back the cookie jar! #CookieJar It's my mission to bring back those memories of a mother baking all day and filling the air with the sweet smell of fresh baked cookies. If done correctly, making your own goodies at home can be delicious and fun at the same time!

In the following pages, I have included a few recipes to help you on your weight loss journey. While reading through these simple recipes, remember that I'm not claiming these snacks are any "healthier" or "better for you" than what you can pick up at the store, a restaurant, or a bakery. I'm just offering you options. Meal prep options. #CookieJar options. Options for you to make on your own in your own kitchen.

Besides that, these recipes are focused on balancing your macros, or altering typical recipes so you have more options for your macro intake. For example, there are two different brownie recipes: a simple tweak to a pre-made box brownie and a low-fat version. Based on the kinds of macros you need to consume, you can choose which recipe fits your needs.

Also, these baked goods are meant to act as protein sources other than the obvious options of meat, beans, and peanut butter. So instead of eating a cookie or a brownie that's high in carbohydrates and fat, you have other options that are a little more balanced macro-wise, increasing your protein intake, while still appeasing your sweet tooth.

Some recipes are tastier than others, but feel free to try them all, making any personal adjustments necessary.

Banana Pancakes

Ingredients

2 ripe bananas
2 scoops whey protein powder

3 Tbsp all-purpose flour
½ teaspoon baking powder

Procedure

1. Beat bananas until soft with electric mixer or food processor. Note: the more ripe the banana, the more moist your pancakes will be.

2. Add protein and mix with mixer or processor until fully incorporated into bananas.

3. Add flour and baking powder. Hand mix with wooden spoon, scrape sides with spatula. Do not overmix.

4. Preheat griddle to 350°F. Spray with non-stick cooking oil.

5. Spoon batter onto griddle.

6. Cook on one side for 60 seconds or until noticeable bubbles appear. Flip and cook on other side for another minute.

7. Remove from griddle, and serve with syrup and your favorite toppings.

*toppings add additional caloric content

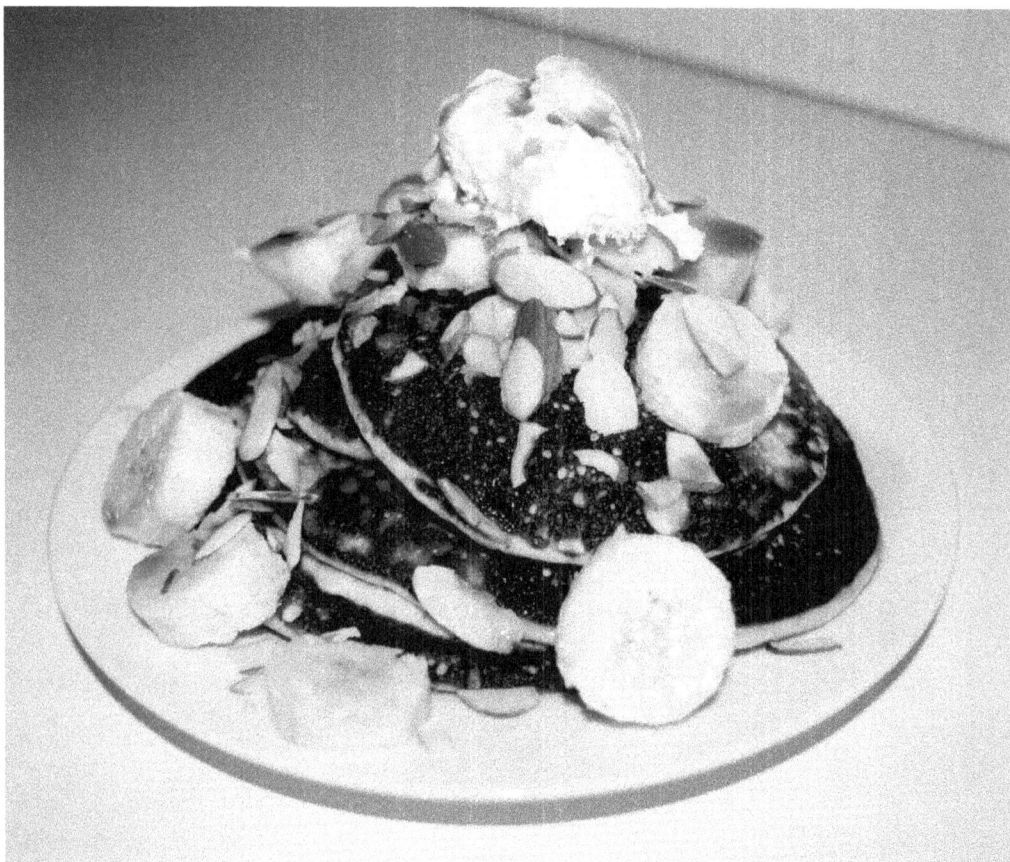

Use pumpkin puree or cooked sweet potatoes for a different flavor pancake!

Approximate Nutrition Facts	
Recipe makes 6 pancakes	
Serving size 1 pancake	
Calories per serving 91	
Fat per serving	0 g
Carbohydrate per serving	14 g
Protein per serving	9 g

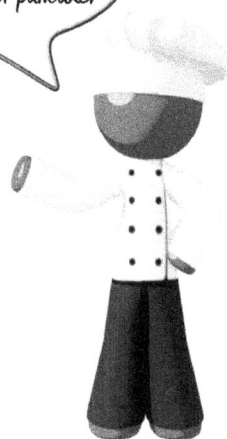

Chocolate Protein Waffles

Ingredients

1 cup Hungry Jack Fluffy pancake mix   1 cup water
1 scoop chocolate whey protein powder   2 Tbsp cocoa powder

Procedure

1. Add all ingredients to a bowl. Whisk together.

2. Some clumps are expected in mixture. Scrape sides with spatula.

3. Preheat waffle iron. Spray with non-stick cooking oil.

4. Spoon batter onto waffle iron. Cook until desired darkness.

5. Remove from waffle iron, and serve with your favorite toppings.

*toppings add additional caloric content

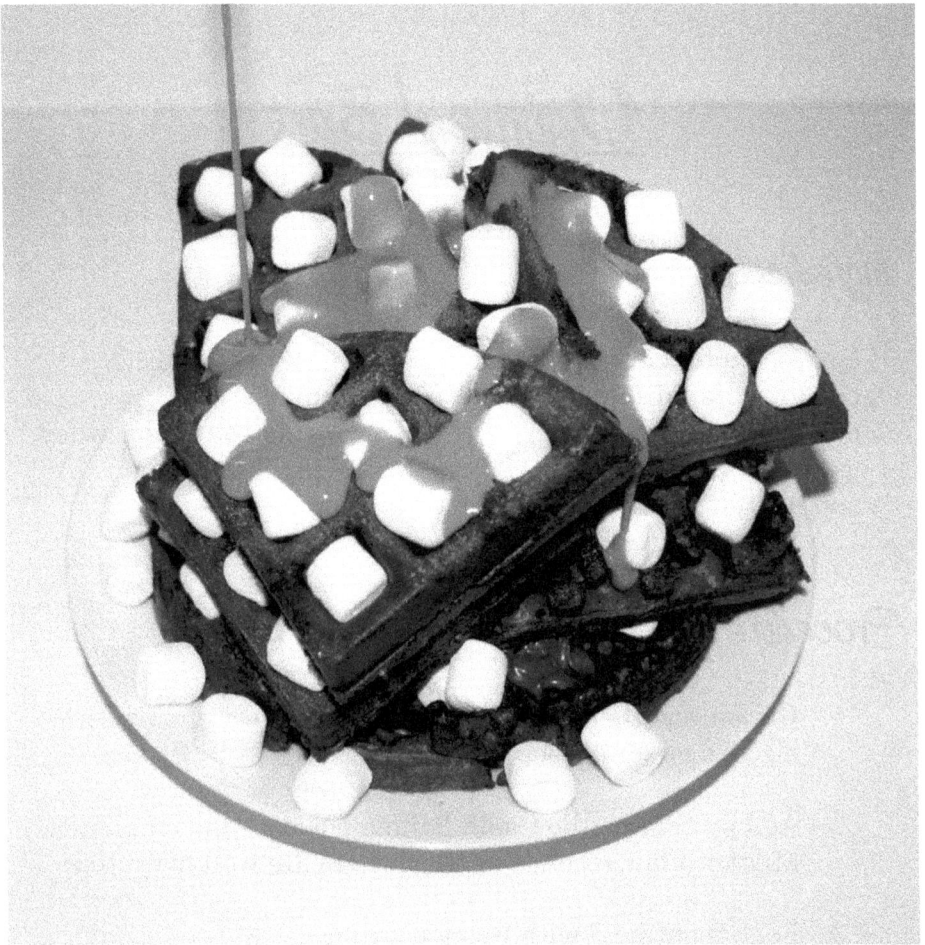

Use the same recipe on the griddle and make chocolate pancakes instead!

Approximate Nutrition Facts	
Recipe makes 3 waffles	
Serving size 1 waffle	
Calories per serving 170	
Fat per serving	2 g
Carbohydrate per serving	28 g
Protein per serving	11 g

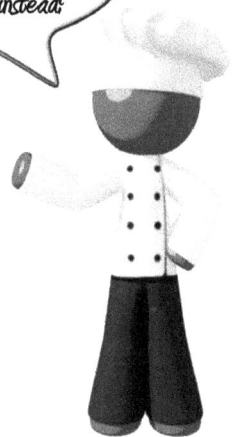

Oatmeal Bars

Ingredients

¼ cup coconut oil or vegetable oil
½ cup granulated sugar
½ cup whey protein powder
1 egg white
¼ cup non-fat plain Greek yogurt

1¼ cup oatmeal
pinch salt
pinch baking powder
pinch cinnamon

Procedure

1. Cream together oil, sugar, egg white, and yogurt with electric mixer or food processor.

2. Add protein powder, salt, baking powder, and cinnamon. Mix for a few seconds until powders are well hydrated.

3. Fold in oatmeal with wooden spoon.

4. Spray 8x8 pan with non-stick cooking oil.

5. Pour mix into pan and spread out evenly with spatula.

6. Bake in preheated oven at 350ºF for 25 minutes.

7. Let cool before cutting into even-sized bars.

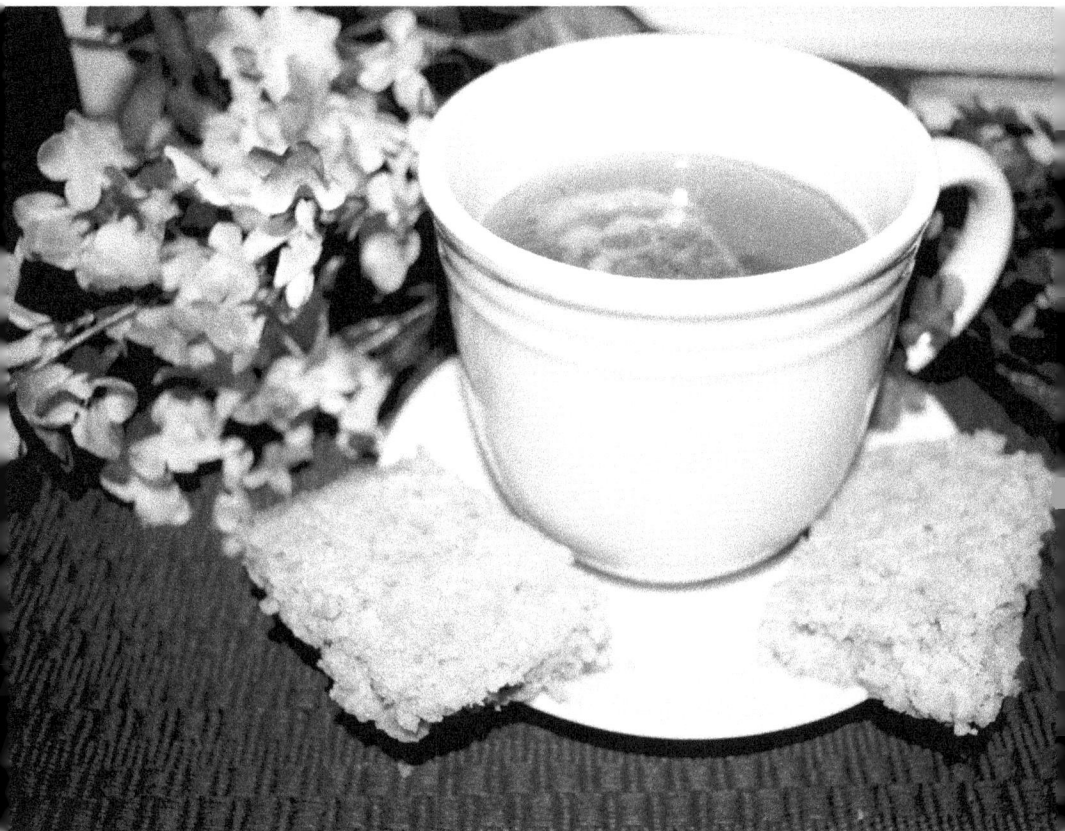

These bars are perfect
served plain
with a side of tea!

Approximate Nutrition Facts	
Recipe makes 9 bars	
Serving size 1 bar	
Calories per serving 167	
Fat per serving	7 g
Carbohydrate per serving	19 g
Protein per serving	7 g

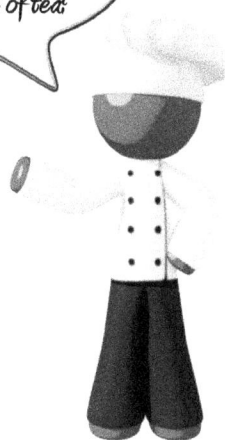

Merengue Drops

Ingredients

3 egg whites
1 tsp vanilla

¼ cup white granulated sugar
2 drops food coloring

Procedure

1. Separate whites from yolks. Do not use liquid egg whites.

2. Beat egg whites with electric mixer until foam forms.

3. Add white sugar one tablespoon at a time to egg whites while beating to maintain foam.

4. Once half the sugar has been mixed with the egg whites, add vanilla. Add a few drops of food coloring to your liking.

5. Finish addition of sugar one tablespoon at a time while continuing to beat with mixer.

6. Cover baking sheet with parchment paper.

7. Fill the mixture into a piping bag to pipe unique shaped drops, or spoon tablespoons of the mix onto baking sheet.

8. Bake at 225°F for 1.5 hours. If oven is too hot, drops will not stay white but will brown instead.

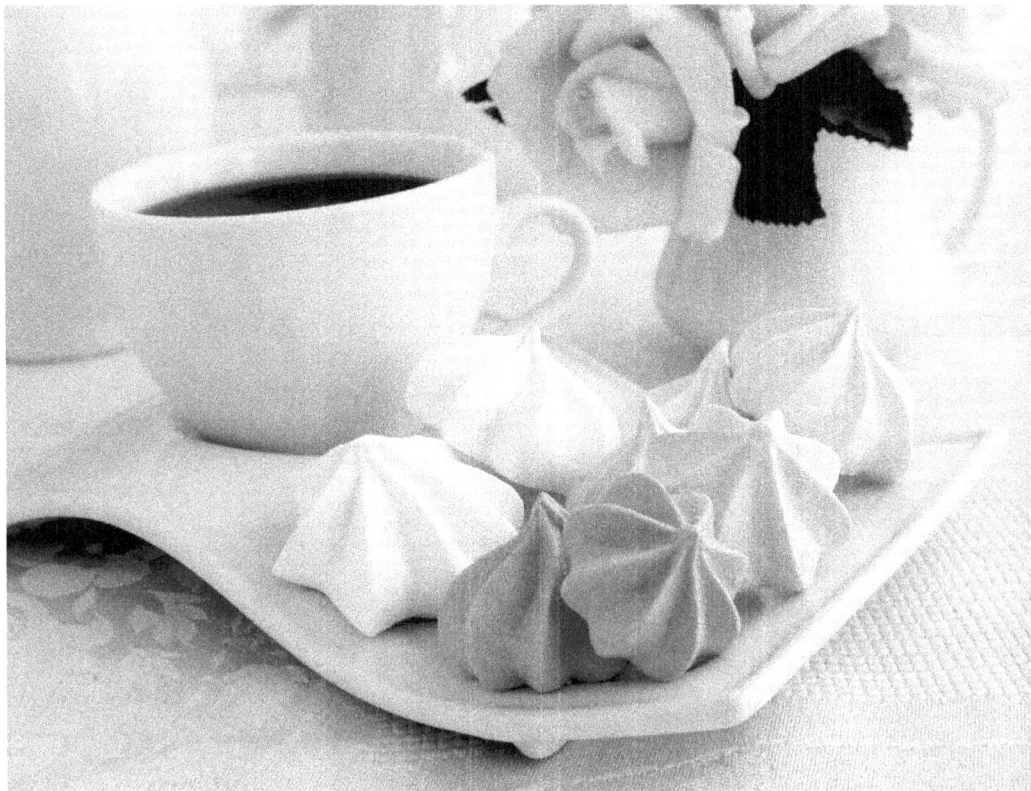

Using different piping methods will give unique shapes to the drops.

Approximate Nutrition Facts	
Recipe makes 24 drops	
Serving size 6 drops	
Calories per serving 61	
Fat per serving	0 g
Carbohydrate per serving	12 g
Protein per serving	3 g

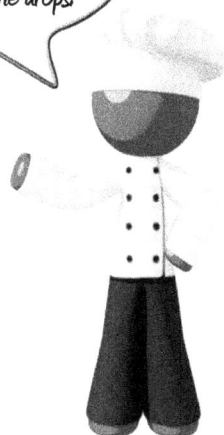

Chocolate Avocado Pie

Ingredients

1.5 scoops whey protein powder

1 cup water

$^3/_4$ cup white granulated sugar

3 Tbsp cocoa powder

1.5 Hass avocado

1 egg

2 egg whites

Procedure

1. Cream avocado with mixer or food processor.

2. Slowly add sugar to avocado.

3. In separate bowl whip together egg, whites, protein, and water.

4. Add ingredients to avocado, and mix together.

5. Mix in cocoa powder.

6. Pour batter into pie pan with premade crust.

7. Bake for an hour at 375ºF.

8. Pie will rise similar to a soufflé. When removing from the oven, the pie will immediately fall.

9. Allow to cool before topping with whipped cream, and serve!

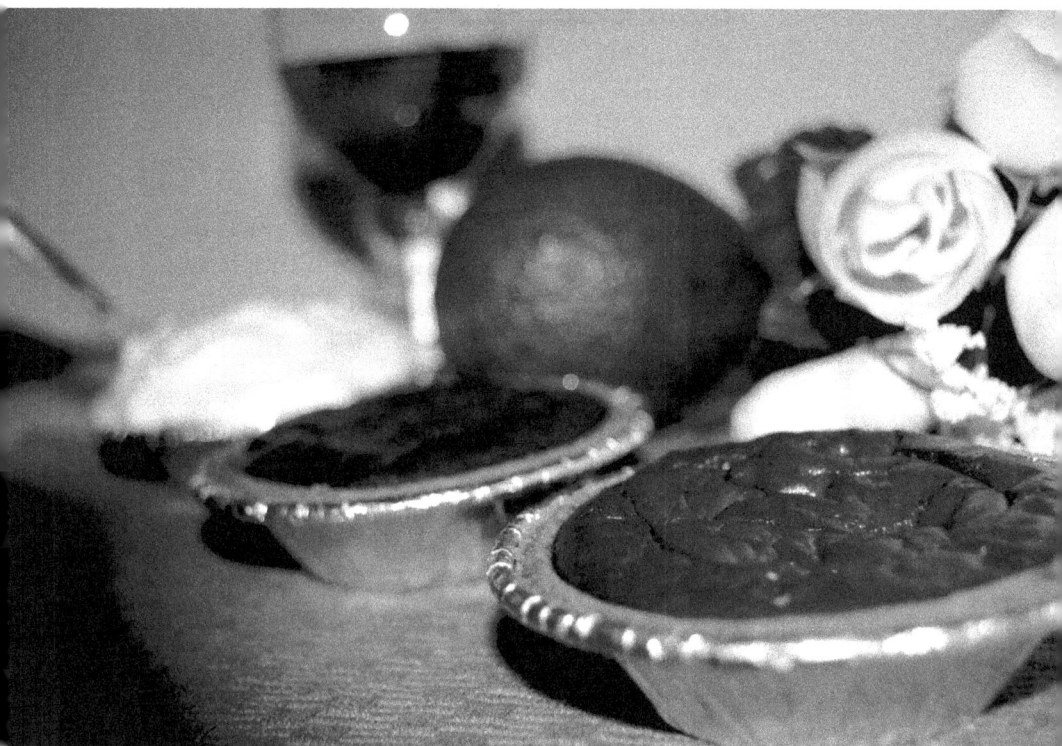

For portion control, bake with mini pie crusts instead— for 45-60 minutes.

Approximate Nutrition Facts	
Recipe makes 1 full pie	
Serving size 1 slice (1/8 of pie)	
Calories per serving 163	
Fat per serving	6 g
Carbohydrate per serving	22 g
Protein per serving	7 g

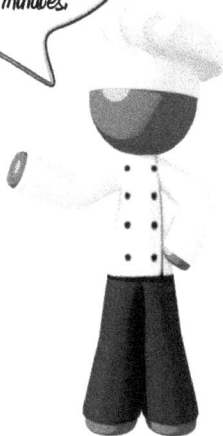

Protein Clusters

Ingredients

2 scoops whey protein powder
½ cup applesauce
3 Tbsp cocoa powder

6 oz low-fat cream cheese
¼ cup sliced almonds
1 cup oatmeal

Procedure

1. Take cream cheese out of the refrigerator to soften.

2. Meanwhile, mix protein powder, applesauce, and cocoa powder together with wooden spoon.

3. If cream cheese is still not soft enough to mix, put in microwave for 5-10 seconds to soften more. Add softened cream cheese to bowl from Step 2. Mix with wooden spoon.

4. Fold in almonds and oatmeal until homogeneous.

5. Place in freezer for 15 minutes to reduce stickiness.

6. Take out of freezer. Scoop the dough with a tablespoon onto cookie sheet.

7. Place in refrigerator to harden.

8. Sprinkle with honey.

*honey and other toppings add additional caloric content

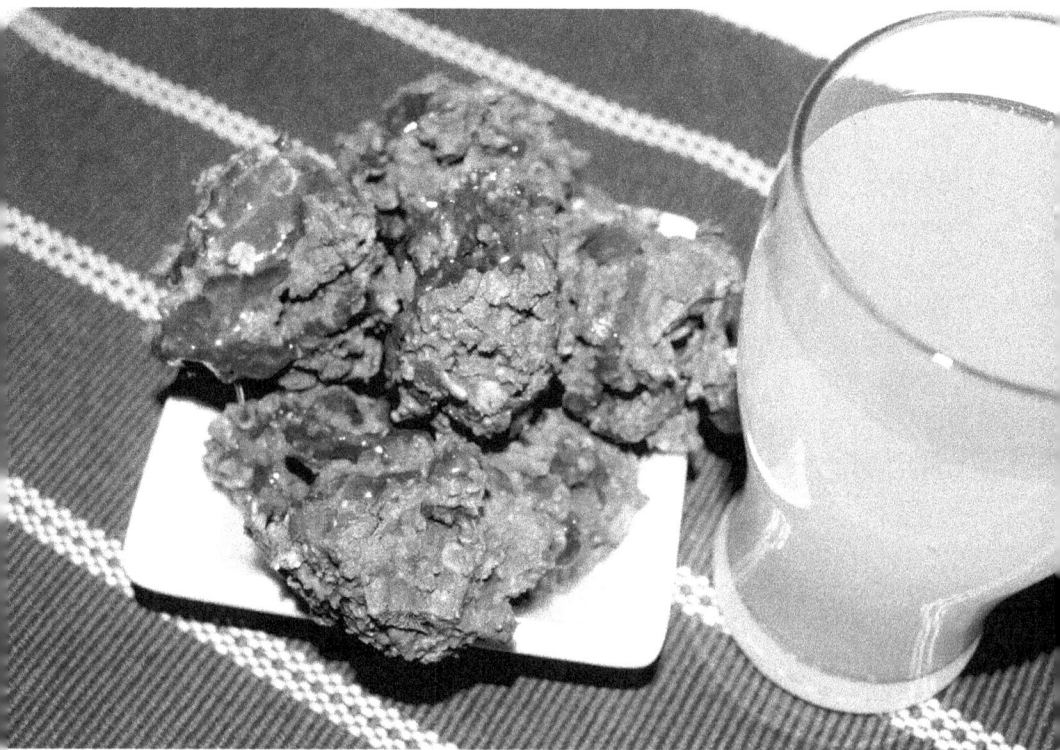

Serve with a nice cold glass of your favorite low-calorie beverage!

Approximate Nutrition Facts	
Recipe makes 12 clusters	
Serving size 1 cluster	
Calories per serving 97	
Fat per serving	5 g
Carbohydrate per serving	8 g
Protein per serving	7 g

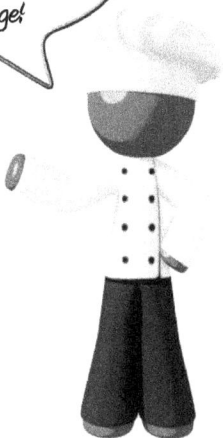

Box Protein Brownies

Ingredients

1 box Pillsbury family size brownie mix
½ cup non-fat plain Greek yogurt
1.5 scoops whey protein powder

2 eggs
½ cup water
⅔ cup vegetable oil

Procedure

1. In medium bowl, combine brownie mix and ingredients as listed on the back of the box (eggs, water, and oil).

2. Add yogurt and protein powder. Mix with wooden spoon for 50 strokes. Do not overmix.

3. Spray 8x8 pan with non-stick cooking oil. Pour mix in pan.

4. Bake in oven for 50 minutes at 350ºF or until toothpick comes out clean.

5. Let cool before cutting into squares.

*toppings add additional caloric content

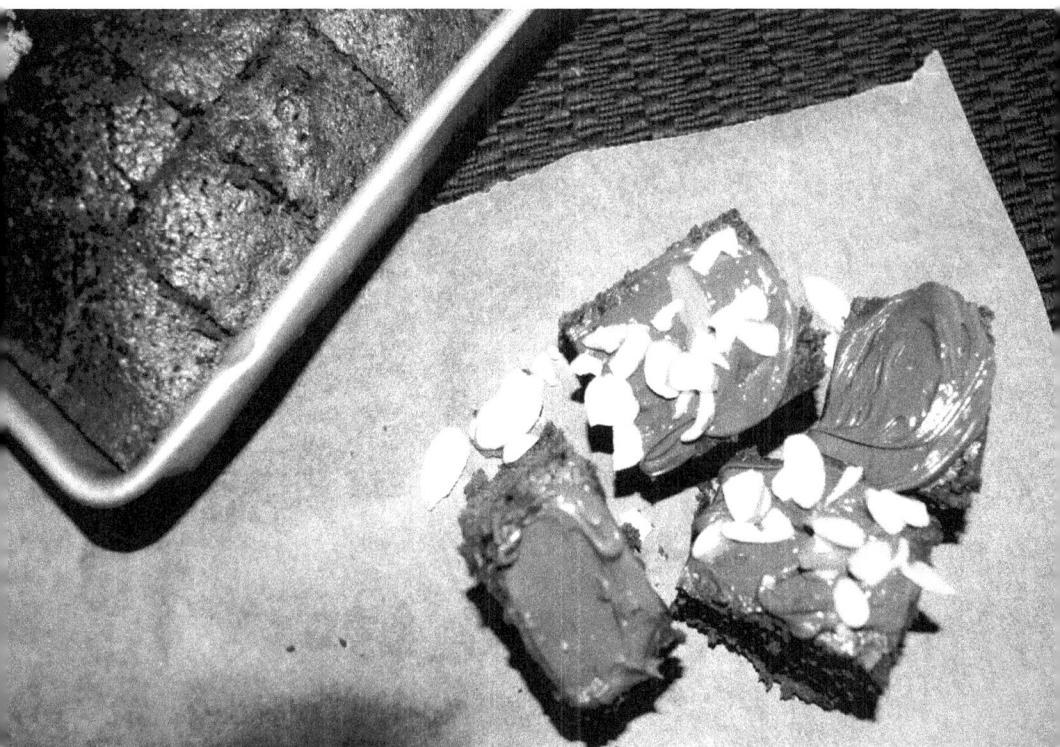

Top these moist brownies with Nutella and almonds for an extra treat!

Approximate Nutrition Facts	
Recipe makes 16 brownies	
Serving size 1 brownie	
Calories per serving 168	
Fat per serving	10 g
Carbohydrate per serving	15 g
Protein per serving	4 g

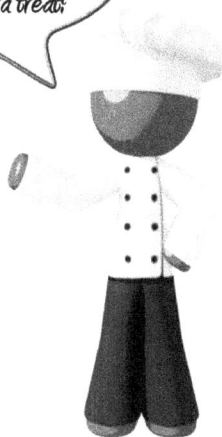

Low-fat Fudge Brownies

Ingredients

1 cup flour
1$^1/_3$ cup dark brown sugar
$^3/_4$ cup cocoa powder
¼ tsp salt
½ tsp baking powder

¾ cup applesauce
½ cup water
2 scoops whey protein powder
4 egg whites
2 tsp vanilla

Procedure

1. Combine all dry ingredients in first column into a large bowl. Mix together with wooden spoon.

2. In a small bowl, combine egg whites and vanilla. Whisk together until uniform mixture.

3. Add applesauce, water, and protein to small bowl. Stir with wooden spoon until protein is hydrated.

4. Add the egg whites mixture to the large bowl. Stir with wooden spoon until well blended (about 50 strokes).

5. Grease and flour two 8x8 pans (one pan for thick brownies).

6. Bake at 350ºF in oven for 1 hour or until toothpick comes out clean (bake longer if using only one pan).

7. Wait until cooled before cutting and serving.

*peanut butter adds additional caloric content

Higher in carbs, but also high in protein, these are fudgy and delectable!

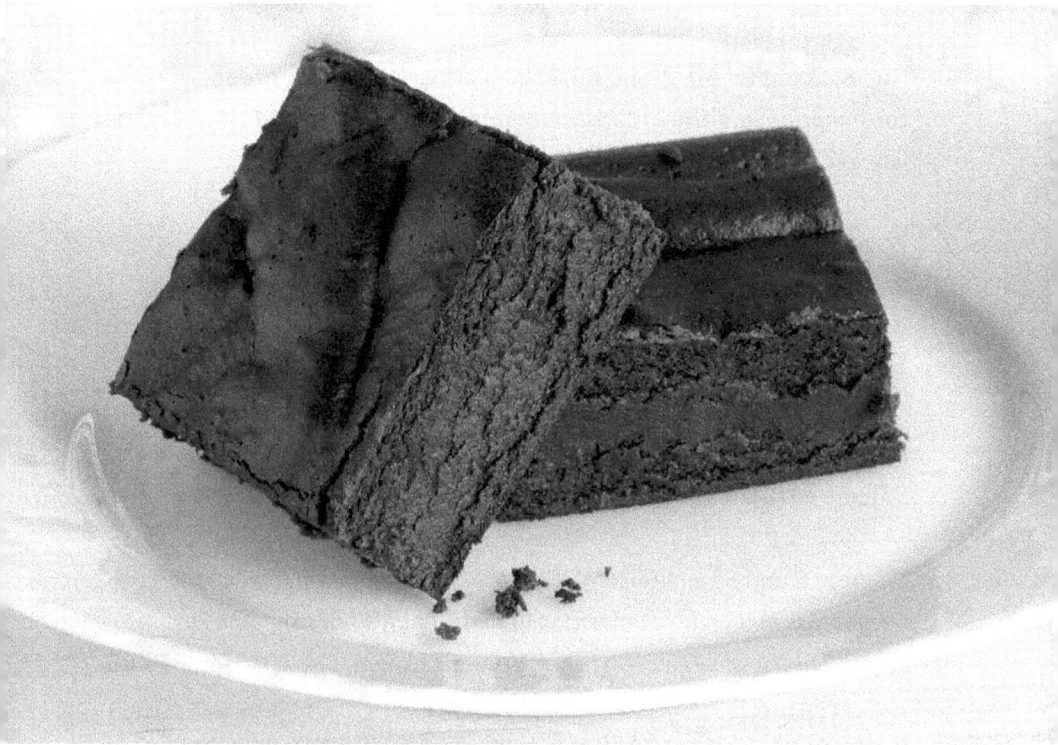

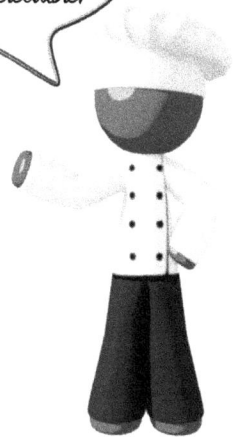

Approximate Nutrition Facts	
Recipe makes 16 brownies	
Serving size 1 brownie	
Calories per serving 123	
Fat per serving	1 g
Carbohydrate per serving	26 g
Protein per serving	5 g

works Cited

1. Hu FB, Stampfer MJ, Rimm EB, *et al. A prospective study of egg consumption and risk of cardiovascular disease in men and women.* JAMA, Volume 281(15), April 1999, pg 1387-94

2. Fernandez ML. *Dietary cholesterol provided by eggs and plasma lipoproteins in healthy populations.* Curr Opin Clin Nutr Metab Care, Volume 9(1), Jan 2006, pg 8-12

3. Nagao K and Yanagita T. *Medium-chain fatty acids: functional lipids for the prevention and treatment of the metabolic syndrome.* Pharmacol Res, Volume 61(3), Mar 2010, pg 208-12

4. Mumme K and Stonehouse W. *Effects of medium-chain triglycerides on weight loss and body composition: a meta-analysis of randomized controlled trials.* J Acad Nutr Diet, Volume 115(2), Feb 2015, pg 249-63

5. Ferdman RA. (2016). *Problem with Parmesan cheese is symbolic of broader issue in American food industry*. Chicago: Chicago Tribune. Retrieved February 18, 2016 from, http://www.chicagotribune.com/business/ct-wood-parmesan-cheese-food-industry-problems-20160217-story.html

6. Freuman TD. (2012). *When nutrition labels lie*. U.S. News & World Report Health. Retrieved February 18, 2016 from, http://health.usnews.com/health-news/blogs/eat-run/2012/ 08/21/when-nutrition-labels-lie

7. Silverglade B and Heller IR. (2010). *Food labeling chaos, the case for reform*. Washington, D.C.: Center for Science in the Public Interest. Retrieved February 18, 2016 from, https://www.cspinet.org/new/pdf/food_labeling_chaos_report.pdf

8. Loftware. *Food & beverage labeling facts.* Portsmouth, NH: Loftware. Retrieved February 18, 2016 from, http://www.loftware.com/resources/Industry_Data_Sheets/FoodandBeverage_dataSheet.pdf

9. Tandel KR. *Sugar substitutes: health controversy over perceived benefits.* J Pharmacol Pharmacother, Volume 2(4), Oct-Dec 2011, pg 236–43.

10. Zwillich T. (2007). *Aspartame safety study stirs emotions.* WebMD. Retrieved February 18, 2016 from, http://www.webmd.com/diet/20070626/aspartame-safety-study-stirs-emotions

11. Simon H and Zieve D. (2016). *Diabetes diet.* Baltimore, MD: University of Maryland Medical Center. Retrieved February 18, 2016 from, http://umm.edu/health/medical/reports/articles/diabetes-diet

12. Mayo Clinic. (2015). *Possible health benefits of sugar alcohols.* Mayo Foundation for Medical Education and Research. Retrieved February 18, 2016 from, http://www.mayoclinic.org/healthy-lifestyle/nutrition-and-healthy-eating/in-depth/artificial-sweeteners/art-20046936?pg=2

13. Trock BJ, Hilakivi-Clarke L, and Clarke R. *Meta-analysis of soy intake and breast cancer risk.* JNCI J Natl Cancer Inst, Volume 98(7), Apr 2006, pg 459-71

14. Kurzer MS. *Hormonal effects of soy in premenopausal women and men.* J Nutr, Volume 132(3), Mar 2002, pg 570S-573S

15. Thornton J. (2009). *Is this the most dangerous food for men?* Men's Health. Retrieved February 18, 2016 from, http://www.menshealth.com/nutrition/soys-negative-effects

16. Zelman KM. (2008). *6 reasons to drink water.* WebMD. Retrieved February 18, 2016 from, http://www.webmd.com/diet/6-reasons-to-drink-water?page=1

17. Mayo Clinic. (2016). *Dietary fats: know which types to choose.* Mayo Foundation for Medical Education and Research. Retrieved February 18, 2016 from, http://www.mayoclinic.org/healthy-lifestyle/nutrition-and-healthy-eating/in-depth/fat/art-20045550

18. U.S. Food and Drug Administration. (2013). Guidance for industry: a food labeling *guide (14. Appendix F: calculate the percent daily value for the appropriate nutrients).* Silver Spring, MD: FDA. Retrieved February 18, 2016 from, http://www.fda.gov/Food/GuidanceRegulation/GuidanceDocumentsRegulatoryInformation/LabelingNutrition/ucm064928.htm

19. Gallagher J. (2015). *Low-fat diets 'better than cutting carbs' for weight loss.* BBC News. Retrieved February 18, 2016 from, http://www.bbc.com/news/health-33905745

Meal tracking worksheet

Column A	Column B		Column C		Column D
Food	**# servings**		**Calories per serving**		**Total Calories (Columns B*C)**
ex. pizza	*2 slices*	x	*350 per slice*	=	*700*
		x		=	
		x		=	
		x		=	
		x		=	
		x		=	
		x		=	
		x		=	
		x		=	
		x		=	
		x		=	
		x		=	
		x		=	

Total calories = _____

Meal tracking worksheet

Column A	Column B		Column C		Column D
Food	**# servings**		**Calories per serving**		**Total Calories (Columns B*C)**
ex. pizza	*2 slices*	x	*350 per slice*	=	*700*
		x		=	
		x		=	
		x		=	
		x		=	
		x		=	
		x		=	
		x		=	
		x		=	
		x		=	
		x		=	
		x		=	
		x		=	

Total calories = _____

Meal tracking worksheet

Column A	Column B		Column C		Column D
Food	**# servings**		**Calories per serving**		**Total Calories (Columns B*C)**
ex. pizza	*2 slices*	x	*350 per slice*	=	*700*
		x		=	
		x		=	
		x		=	
		x		=	
		x		=	
		x		=	
		x		=	
		x		=	
		x		=	
		x		=	
		x		=	
		x		=	

Total calories = _____

Meal tracking worksheet

Column A	Column B		Column C		Column D
Food	**# servings**		**Calories per serving**		**Total Calories (Columns B*C)**
ex. pizza	2 slices	x	350 per slice	=	700
		x		=	
		x		=	
		x		=	
		x		=	
		x		=	
		x		=	
		x		=	
		x		=	
		x		=	
		x		=	
		x		=	
		x		=	

Total calories = _____

Meal tracking worksheet

Column A	Column B		Column C		Column D
Food	# servings		Calories per serving		Total Calories (Columns B*C)
ex. pizza	2 slices	x	350 per slice	=	700
		x		=	
		x		=	
		x		=	
		x		=	
		x		=	
		x		=	
		x		=	
		x		=	
		x		=	
		x		=	
		x		=	
		x		=	

Total calories = _____

Meal tracking worksheet

Column A	Column B		Column C		Column D
Food	**# servings**		**Calories per serving**		**Total Calories (Columns B*C)**
ex. pizza	*2 slices*	x	*350 per slice*	=	*700*
		x		=	
		x		=	
		x		=	
		x		=	
		x		=	
		x		=	
		x		=	
		x		=	
		x		=	
		x		=	
		x		=	
		x		=	

Total calories = _____

Professor Cookie

coming to a location near you!

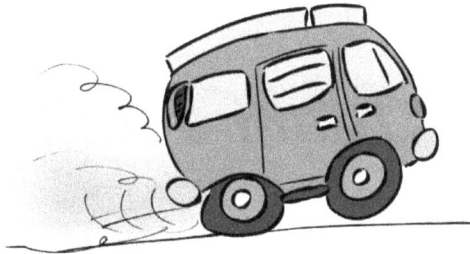

Join the Professor
at a gym or school auditorium near you
for an informational presentation
about the food you eat!

**Send an email to
JunkFoodFit@gmail.com
for more information today!**

www·JunkFoodFit·com

www.ingramcontent.com/pod-product-compliance
Lightning Source LLC
Chambersburg PA
CBHW060604200326
41521CB00007B/656